Young for Life

The Easy NO-DIET, NO-SWEAT Plan to Look and Feel 10 YEARS YOUNGER

Marilyn Diamond

and

Dr. Donald "Rock" Schnell

RODALE.

For our beloved children and grandchildren

Rodale books may be purchased for business or promotional use or for special sales. For information, please write to:
Special Markets Department, Rodale Inc., 733 Third Avenue, New York, NY 10017

Printed in the United States of America
Rodale Inc. makes every effort to use acid-free ♾, recycled paper ♻.

Book design by Elizabeth Neal

Library of Congress Cataloging-in-Publication Data is on file with the publisher.

ISBN: 978–1–60961–542–0 hardcover

Distributed to the trade by Macmillan

2   4   6   8   10   9   7   5   3   1   hardcover

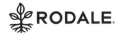

We inspire and enable people to improve their lives and the world around them.
rodalebooks.com

Contents

PART THREE
THE ANABOLIC FOODS

PART SEVEN
MAKING OUR SYSTEM WORK IN YOUR LIFE

Foreword

As a traditionally trained board-certified cardiologist, I have always been skeptical of unproven ideas. My natural scientific skepticism has made me very wary of health claims through the years. For example, the so-called scientific data that came out years ago suggesting that eating red meat or eggs could somehow be bad for us seemed questionable to me, particularly because those foods have been a staple of the diets of successful societies for thousands of years. By looking at people like Jack LaLanne, with all of his muscularity, who reached 96 years old in a highly functional condition, it seemed obvious to me that eating carrot sticks and running numerous marathons were not necessarily the keys to longevity. Jack knew the importance of strength training and protein in the diet (although he shunned meat for fish in his later years).

Muscularity, vitality, sensuality, and ultimately the pursuit of youth all appear to be the new direction that the scientific community—myself included—has begun to pursue for our patients and ourselves. That is precisely why I feel this book has the power to change so many lives.

The ideas presented here are not only intuitive to most, but many are also substantiated by significant research. Furthermore, authors Marilyn Diamond and Dr. Donald "Rock" Schnell practice what they preach. Only recently has the mainstream medical community become humbled by doctors and nutritionists flip-flopping over fundamental ideas surrounding carbohydrates versus fats, recalled drugs we once thought to be wonder medicines, and questioned overuse of certain medical procedures. In fact, the scientific community has only recently endorsed many of the nutrients discussed in this book as being highly beneficial. Finally, now that we understand that human hormones tend to deplete themselves over the natural course of our life span (and often starting in our late twenties), we are beginning to study and employ methods to maintain their important effects. The authors of this book have recognized that sobering fact and have utilized their expertise, abundant research, and the available scientific data to present a practical program to extend your body's ability to achieve its full potential.

Young for Life gets back to basics in a powerfully insightful way, and it reminds us just how wonderful a machine is the optimally nourished human body. It also offers tools to maximize your body-machine. The authors provide easy-to-follow techniques for effective yet moderate exercise, an intuitive and delicious eating plan, and useful advice about embracing our sexuality.

Our bodies are designed to give us many years of strength, vitality, and pleasure. It seems that only when we embrace lifestyles that are counterproductive to the body's natural design do we lessen the quality and length of our life span. My own observations have shown that the current fads of extreme diets and excessive and destructive exercise leave many of my patients frustrated and less than fulfilled. I hope that they, and you, will experience the passion for life and all of its bounty that Marilyn and Rock express in this book and take from me, their physician and friend, the encouragement to begin truly *living again!*

Ariel Soffer, MD

Ariel Soffer, MD, is board certified in cardiovascular disease and is a prevention-oriented cardiologist in Miami, Florida. His internship and residency training was at Cedars-Sinai Medical Center, UCLA. He is an associate clinical professor of medicine at Florida International University and Nova Southeastern University Medical Schools. He is a frequent scientific contributor to *Life Extension* magazine, *Endovascular Today*, and many other peer-reviewed scientific journals, as well as a frequent medical expert on ABC, CBS, NBC, and Fox News programs.

Marilyn
DIAMOND

Last week I had a massage with a new therapist who knew nothing about me. It was a thorough deep-tissue treatment of my entire body. At the end of the massage, I suddenly had the impulse to ask, "How old do you think I am, Kyle?"

His response came quickly: "Oh, not older than thirty-five."

I have a son who's 45!

The fact is people often say that I look far younger than I am. What matters more to me is to help you see that you, too, can look and feel years younger.

The way I look today is the result of following the secrets I want to share with you in this book. In one workout, I can do multiple sets of squats, deadlifts, and pushups with no problem in record time, because my program has taught me how to do the exercises efficiently. I can work out at the gym, but most often I work out in my home office. This way, even while working, I can repeat my routine throughout the day.

I wasn't always as strong as I am today. In fact, I started in 2009 with just a basic 6-second technique of muscle contraction, which you'll read about in this book. It's the foundation of shaping sexy muscle. This is the secret that most people need to learn today, and I'm so excited to be able to share it. Using this technique, I can tone my abs and shoulders while I'm sitting at my computer. I can tone my buns standing in line at the supermarket or waiting for an elevator. I know what to do, and I want you to know what to do, because as I write this to you, I believe that this is the time for you to give up convenience foods and to become serious about convenience exercise.

At 69, I'm living my dream of remaining youthful without paying any attention to my age.

Twenty-seven years ago, I was on a national tour, crisscrossing the country for presentations and talk show appearances to share the principles I'd developed for my bestselling book *Fit for Life*. But today, I can honestly report that I am in *far* better condition *now* than I ever was back then—physically, mentally, and *spiritually*.

You may be in your twenties, thirties, forties, or fifties. You may be my age or older, and if so, great! No matter your age, if you are the kind of person who wants to sail through life in a truly fit body, this is your book. If you want to feel happy and confident about your health so you can flirt confidently with life's pleasures and eagerly take on life's challenges, this book is for you. It's for anyone who wants to experience the mind-blowing freedom that comes when your body reaches its pinnacle of performance and a powerful magnetism of attraction takes over in your life. That's when all good things start to happen.

I wanted this level of magical vitality "someday" when I was 31, and the seed of this book began to germinate. I've spent the past 37 years searching to make that "someday" happen. The fact is, "someday is here," and now you are in possession of some very powerful solutions for staying young.

LOVE TO THE RESCUE

I'm not writing this book on my own. I'm working with my incredibly knowledgeable husband and partner of 20 years, the "dream weaver" I knew would someday find me. I wanted to stay young, so that when the soul mate I was looking for arrived, I would be the girl of his dreams, too.

I met Donald Schnell on July 29, 1992, 4 months after my not-so-fit-for-life marriage imploded. He found me worn out and devastated. Much later, he confessed that when he first saw me, he asked himself, "Who's been stomping my sunflower?"

I gave everything I had to the *Fit for Life* years, and, for the sake of my children and my audience, I walked away when there was almost nothing left of me. Donald and I began a wonderful union 4 years later, and we both wept with joy when we took our wedding vows. From that day on, because we wanted as many young and vital years as possible together, we have made it our focus to find the unknown secrets to prevent and reverse the symptoms of premature aging.

My partner today has training and a lifetime of research and experience in nutrition, psychology, effective ways to strengthen the body with or without equipment, and effective ways to strengthen and harness the mind and use its powers to stay youthful.

After military service, he completed his bachelor's degree in elementary education at Arizona State University and his master's of science in computer education at Nova Southeastern University. He taught in elementary and middle schools for 10 years, closing the last few years of his teaching career with the assignment to "rescue" the most difficult students, which allowed him to bring many failing students to advanced levels of achievement. Even today, his former students still write to him.

A serious automobile accident in 1985 left Donald with a broken shoulder held together by a large metal pin. Fearing that he might have to give up his lifelong passion for weight training and fitness, he moved on to three years of graduate study at Palmer College of Chiropractic. His goal was to master the musculoskeletal system, anatomy, physiology, biochemistry, and nutrition so that he could rehabilitate himself and live in a strong body for the rest of his life and help others achieve the same goals. He then transferred his graduate study credits at Palmer and completed his doctorate in clinical hypnotherapy at the American Institute of Hypnotherapy in Irvine, California.

My coauthor is a powerful guide and expert in the many ways we can shape the mind and body for optimal achievement in life. From 1992 to 1998, we coauthored several books and online courses. From 1998 to 2008, we taught much of this system together in seminars we called "The Power of Love." If you want to know how to feel younger at any age, Donald is your resource. Like me, he has dedicated his entire life to exploring the information we are about to share with you. We have both tested and refined the elements of this approach to nutrition and exercise for a long time to prove to ourselves that we have found what truly works.

When I began to re-create the new Marilyn from the worn-out ruins of the old, I found out through trial and error that it's easier than you could ever believe to be exceedingly youthful, healthy, and happy. You might not think that would be possible since so many "experts" are constantly contradicting one another, and nobody seems to be making much progress. They mean well, but they aren't making it any easier for you.

The secrets I will share are so natural and basic they are poised to burst forth like a fountain of youth when you release them. My goal is to help you let this fountain flow once and for all. I am a living example that you can turn up the flame on your energy at any age and participate in life on a new level of adventure and excitement.

YOUNG ON THE INSIDE

In the spring of 2012, I had my yearly physical exam. My cardiologist told me my lab results were excellent. My blood pressure is normally around 118 over 60. My hormones are in great shape. My blood sugar is normal. My resting pulse is around 50. My HDL cholesterol is healthfully high. I have a great appetite and no problem with digestion, and I most often sleep like a baby. I take my yearly exams, but other than that, I spend virtually no time in doctor's waiting rooms. I have so much energy that I work and play longer and harder than I did 10 years ago. I'm more resourceful, inventive, and motivated as well. I often feel that I have wings on my feet and I'm flying, because I feel so young and excited about the potential I still have to help others!

What good is living if we can't fully enjoy our lives and get out of the rut of thinking that life has to be a hardship? This program gives you fighting fire to see that all of life's challenges are simply opportunities to grow so that we can turn challenges into exciting possibilities. I know from experience that if you choose the direction Dr. Rock and I are suggesting, you'll discover a new level of vitality that creates a turning point in your life.

I DON'T DIET; YOU WON'T EITHER

To be in the best shape of your life *you have to eat!* I eat a greater variety of food now than I've eaten in 30 years. You must eat sufficient quantities of the right foods, *not the wrong foods,* every 3 to 4 hours to keep your blood sugar stable and avoid cravings. There are certain foods I eat and certain foods I don't eat. I've learned that mealtime should not be a random or mindless exercise. It takes planning.

Certain foods contain the nutrients that make us young and energetic, and many others contain the nutrients that slow us down and age us. Neither you nor I should have any interest in the latter! But when you find out what the first group is, you're going to be quite surprised. You get to eat a wide variety of really tasty food on this program!

Nutrients are the molecules that make up the very structure of our bodies. Everything exciting in health today is happening at the molecular level. As scientists test and verify their hypotheses on the effect of nutrients, then retest and duplicate results, they are finding that it all boils down to what you eat and how active you are. With advanced imaging techniques, scientists can watch nerves, DNA, and mitochondria as they thrive or are under siege, whichever the case may be, because of certain lifestyle choices. They can see what happens with every bite of food you take. They can see the effect of exercise and stress on your DNA or on the life of a cancer cell. You can take advantage of what they are seeing and reporting, and be in *complete control* of how young you will feel or how fast you will age! How will you achieve this? Will you do yoga, take a long walk, or do Pilates? Will you consume green juice and fruit or some dark chocolate? A soy protein shake? A salad and a chicken breast? The answers are in this book, and they may surprise you.

With an understanding of the power of nutrients in your body, your quest going forward is to be *anabolic*. This word means the metabolic process of building up your body's tissues and organs. And it's very important to recapturing your youth and staying young in body and mind. (We will discuss anabolism in greater detail later on.)

Anabolic! Anabolism! Remember these key words for a new level of achievement in remaining youthful and healthy. Just this one concept allowed me to remove myself from the list of 30 million prematurely aging "skinny-fat" Americans who are now among the 170 million people in our country who are part of the obesity epidemic.

THE SILENT EPIDEMIC

As a leading spokeswoman for diet and health since 1985, I have brought to my readers the revolutionary *Fit for Life* lifestyle, based on eating large quantities of fresh fruits and vegetables. Mine was a breakthrough concept that for the first time connected diet to health for a mainstream audience. This is my greatest achievement to date, because at that time, traditional medicine was in complete opposition to the idea that our food choices could actually improve our health. But I fought for you and held my ground because I'd been living my system of eating mostly fruits and vegetables for over a decade, and I knew I was right. My program created greater energy and radiance, and although the traditional medical community didn't accept it, the entertainment community did. As they hosted talk shows or walked the red carpet, dozens of actors, models, television personalities, and fashion designers told stories about their own success with *Fit for Life* to millions of Americans. Within just a few years, the American Heart Association came on board and essentially forced the medical community to accept fresh fruits and vegetables as health foods. A few years later, the surgeon general, backing the notion that you are what you eat, proclaimed that more than 60 percent of diseases can be connected to dietary choices.

Fit for Life was part of my search for the kind of body I'm promising you in this book. It was the part that allowed me to be fashionably thin, but not toned. It was the part that I now realize was not a long-term solution. You see, *Fit for Life* lacked key pieces of information that could not easily be found in the years before we had the Internet to access journals, forums, and the blogs of experts. It was a good step, but just one step along the way. Obviously, *Fit for Life* was pioneering work, and not my end point. It had to evolve into something truer and greater.

I was a pioneer in the raw food, vegetarian, and vegan movements. Few people my age have followed those lifestyles for as long as I did. I'm speaking out in this book because we should all be up front about our experiences and our choices. After nearly 20 years of following a low-protein diet (low in both quantity and quality of protein), I was dangerously protein deficient. I also had a decades-long passion for aerobic exercise, and these two choices combined to create a serious condition I knew nothing about. I became what's called skinny-fat.

Overweight obesity is not ideal. Neither is skinny-fat obesity! The problem that creates both conditions is hidden in misinformation. The problem in both is a muscle-to-fat ratio that is out of balance. Fortunately, groundbreaking research in diet and exercise removed my name from the list of millions who are suffering from the various symptoms of this epidemic problem.

I was ultimately immobilized by this condition, an early-onset symptom of aging. I was so skinny-fat, so emaciated, that I lost the important lean muscle tissue I needed to cushion my bones and protect my nerves. I was underweight and nutrient deficient, but, like most people, I just succumbed to the fact that, at age 60, I would just have to cope with it and this was a natural part of the aging process. I lived in terror of chronic nerve compression in my neck that shot lightning bolts of pain into my head, down my spine, and down my arms. When this happened, it was as if everything stopped momentarily. My circulation, my respiratory system, my very life blinked off for a moment. And then, nausea would overcome me, and weakness, which lasted for hours.

Now, don't be alarmed or confused. I was not suffering from some rare neurological disorder. I had a common lifestyle deficiency caused by my diet and exercise routine.

If you think something is bad for you (like butter), hold on, because I'm going to show you it's probably better for you than you can possibly imagine. I have personally experienced the symptoms of the two silent epidemics that are killing us today, so I can warn you about them. According to the latest research, these epidemics will overwhelm us in the next few generations if we don't do something to stop them now. One is either being sedentary or overdoing cardio to the point that brings about muscle wasting. The second is nutrient deficiencies—literally the underlying cause of nearly every disease. I'm living proof we can stop these epidemics, and we can feel a great deal of fulfillment and fun doing so.

"HEALTHY" AND "HAPPY" ARE CODE WORDS FOR SURVIVAL

I was totally willing to reject the aspects of my 27-year-old *Fit for Life* program that were no longer relevant. I was totally willing to learn that as I aged in such a restrictive program, I'd triggered muscle wasting, nutrient deficiency, and loss of libido. For decades, I had lived on a meatless diet—about 80 percent raw fruits and vegetables. You can imagine my shock when my research uncovered that vegetarians *do not* live longer than the rest of the population and are at the same risk of degenerative diseases.

Thin is in, but it should be out. Thin is not the answer to the obesity crisis. Thin is a *huge* compromise that triggers consequences that now simply must be revealed. The fact is strong is the new sexy. Strength is youth!

Throughout history, it's the strong—not the weak—who carried us through, and they also kept our gene pool going. In this era, with all the dire predictions of the "tsunami of disease" we're facing, survival of the fittest beckons to you to take this message seriously.

I realize that some people will see my position today as a reversal of the lifestyle I once lived and promoted, and that's okay. I am a member of Phi Beta Kappa, the 230-year-old national honor society for the top

1 percent of college graduates. As a member of this society, I have dedicated my life to the principles of freedom of inquiry and liberty of thought and expression. I was raised by one of the greatest molecular biologists of the twentieth century. My father, Bernard L. Horecker, PhD, was the dean of Weill Cornell University Graduate School of Medical Sciences when I was launching my *Fit for Life* research. By birth and upbringing, I am first and foremost a researcher who is searching for the answers that will improve the lives of my readers. The science of 2013 eclipses the science of 1985, for those who are willing to delve into it. I'm here after pulling myself out of extreme pain and rapid decline, because I don't want you going there, making the same mistakes I made. I'm here because I had the courage to break away from the myths that are entrenched in the Western culture of disease.

New things have always come at the beginning of a century that make whatever was going on in the previous century obsolete. This is certainly true in health and fitness, and I want you to be the living proof.

A MESSAGE FROM
Dr.
ROCK

I f you have a pulse and you're paying any attention to the news, you're aware that we're facing a real health crisis in the United States. The forecasts are dire, and it's no mystery that in the next several decades we will witness alarming disease statistics.

• According to a recent report in the *Lancet,* 50 percent of Americans will be obese by 2030. With obesity comes the imbalanced muscle-to-fat ratio that leads to blockages in the brain and the arteries and inadequate secretion of hormones.

- Every 6 seconds an American is diagnosed with diabetes, and during that same 6 seconds, the disease kills one person globally, reports the journal *Diabetes Care.*
- The American Diabetes Association predicts that as many as 44 million Americans will suffer the devastating symptoms and side effects of diabetes by 2034, at a cost of $336 billion.
- American Heart Association statistics show that every 29 seconds an American suffers a coronary event, and just about every 25 seconds someone in the United States dies from one. Approximately one-third (34 percent) of cardiovascular deaths occur before age 75. Almost one out of every four deaths results from cardiovascular disease.
- According to the Centers for Disease Control and Prevention, about half of all Americans will experience some form of mental health problem, such as depression, stress, or anxiety disorder, during their lifetime.
- According to a study in the *Journal of the American Medical Association,* 43 percent of women experience sexual dysfunction.
- Researchers at the State University of New York predict that one out of three Americans will develop cancer, and one of out four males and one out of three females will die of cancer. The National Institutes of Health estimated the 2010 overall annual costs of cancer at $263.8 billion.
- The Alzheimer's Association reports that 5.4 million people have Alzheimer's disease, accounting for an estimated 14.9 million unpaid caregivers and $183 billion in annual costs.

These are frightening statistics. But the whole point Marilyn and I want to make in this book is that it doesn't have to be this way for you. You don't have to be part of these sad statistics. It takes only the right information and the proper application of that information for you to rise above this disease tsunami. Let me tell you a little more about myself so you'll understand my experience, my commitment to your youthful health, and my passion for sharing this information.

MY STORY

I was unexpectedly forced into one of the dire forecasts described above in 2009. I had been feeling unwell for a few months, so I took my usual step and went on a raw food diet to see if I could wipe out any symptoms and put myself back together. Since Marilyn and I were in the process of relocating from California to Florida to spend some time with her aging parents, seeing a doctor wasn't going to happen right away. Not going to see a physician and eating raw food were both mistakes because I began to drop weight very rapidly. Within a few months, *skinny* was an understatement to describe my body. But the problem was much more complicated than this. I was in a vicious cycle of being excessively thirsty all the time and urinating all the time—day and night. I had an insatiable craving for enormous amounts of fruit and would eat half a watermelon, half a dozen oranges, or four bananas in one sitting. I rationalized that I was healing and my body was fruit starved. Frankly, there was so much else to do that I couldn't focus on my own situation.

We spent 2 months in Charlotte, North Carolina, with family. When we reached Florida, I was going from bad to worse. My in-laws were worried. I looked gaunt. Marilyn, too, was alarmed and arranged for me to go through a cardiovascular screening at the local YMCA in a new program being offered to gather statistics about the local population. She had to finagle quite aggressively to get me in right away. Good thing she did. My hemoglobin A1c (HbA1c) blood test, which charts a 3-month average of blood sugar levels, was at the highest level, 11.9, or 1 percentage point from death. The nurses were in a panic. I was rushed to a local primary care physician. On my 55th birthday, February 4, 2009, I was diagnosed with late-onset type 1 diabetes. The doctor immediately put me on Lantus, and overnight I was injecting myself with the insulin. I never thought this would happen to me. I was completely unprepared, and so was Marilyn. My physician explained the very complicated nature of the disease, but to be honest, both Marilyn and I were in shock. It was hard to grasp what had happened to me.

Here's what I did learn: I had the most devastating form of diabetes. Between my life and my death was that bottle of insulin in my refrigerator. My future suddenly held the possibility of limb amputations and blindness. I now had a 76 percent greater risk of heart attack. The biggest odds were against me! But I was in love and I wanted my life with Marilyn; none of this fit my picture. I plunged into depression, and as I followed the recommended dietary guidelines for diabetics, to eat more servings of grain and certain other carbohydrates, my body went from skinny to puffy, like the Pillsbury Doughboy's. Since I had always been muscular, looking like this only added to my depression. I found myself searching for what to do.

Marilyn was at the computer day and night trying to keep our writing going, and suddenly, under the stress of all that was happening to us, she couldn't move her neck. She went to visit her daughter in Virginia to give me a chance to regroup on my own. When she returned, I laid out my plan. I said, "Look, I'm fighting this disease. I'm not going to be its victim. Sweetheart, I'm not going to die young and lose you. I've made up my mind. Since muscle burns sugar out of the blood, I'm going to put on as much muscle as I can."

"I'll do it with you!" she said. "I'll go to the gym and lift weights. I'll eat what you eat. I'll do anything you do and need me to do."

I knew she would react this way, but I was still heartened to have her support and participation. "I've studied the earliest diets used for this disease, from before there was insulin," I explained. "Don't be shocked, but I want to cut all carbs out of my diet. It helped people survive before prescription insulin was available, and that's what I want to try. I'll stay on the insulin, because if I don't, I'm dead. But I'll see what I can do to limit the collateral damage. I'll keep searching for the information that can make a difference."

She stuck with me, and my sweetheart, who was a vegetarian for decades, was now preparing three or four high-protein meals a day. And I was buried in research and searching for more information on how to save us. This search is part of how this book came about.

A short time into this new way of living, a catastrophic family situation took over our lives. New to my condition, I was not yet fully aware of the management of my disease under stress. Stress sends blood sugar through the roof. Even if you are on insulin, stress can send blood sugar to three or four times its normal reading. Suddenly trapped in this family ordeal I couldn't avoid or prevent, I found myself away from home for long periods and without my insulin, which had to be refrigerated. The stress drove my blood sugar so high and my blood became so thick that it stopped my heart. *I had my diabetic heart attack.*

The endocrinologists and cardiologists at the hospital I was admitted to concurred that I had congestive heart failure and cardiomyopathy with an ejection fraction of 32 percent. Ejection fraction is the measurement of the amount of blood that the heart pumps with each beat. My score indicated life-threatening heart failure.

My hospital records told the story, and I went as quickly as I could for a consultation with Ariel Soffer, MD, who verified the results. All my doctors said that my condition would only worsen and that I had a maximum of 5 years to live. They warned me that I could drop dead at any time because a second heart attack would undoubtedly prove fatal.

I looked into Marilyn's beautiful green eyes, which had darkened from lack of sleep, her face gaunt with worry. I vowed for the second time in less than a year that I would not let death take me. I resolved to fight back harder than I'd ever fought in my life, with all my mental and physical power.

With Marilyn fully engaged in my struggle, I designed an advanced program of nutrition and power-lifting exercise for myself, building on the research that we already had in progress. Within 2 years, I succeeded in lowering my blood sugar enough to prevent or reverse the effects of type 1 diabetes, including peripheral neuropathy, retinopathy, loss of libido, and increased risk of heart attack.

As for the low ejection fraction that I was warned would only worsen, I took care of that as well. When I showed up for retesting with Dr. Soffer, I had put on 30 pounds of lean muscle. That 30 pounds of careful muscle development seemed to have assisted my heart to become 30 percent stronger. My ejection fraction had risen from 32 to 58 percent. Dr. Soffer was so surprised by the results of my tests that he repeated them immediately, and then returned to the exam room where Marilyn and I were waiting.

Shaking his head in disbelief, he said, "This just doesn't happen, Rock. It's not in the textbooks. The ejection fraction always declines. If I believed in miracles, I would say this would have to be one."

My HbA1c blood sugar reading came next, and I succeeded there as well. From the exercise, diet, and supplements I'd discovered, I'd lowered it from 11.9 in February 2009—that "write your will" level—to 5.5 in August 2011. My physician, Dr. Varney, said, "Your blood sugar is lower than mine, and technically, at this point, you're managing your diabetes to the level of a nondiabetic. You can slowly cut your insulin down, and you should so that you don't go hypoglycemic. You might actually be making some insulin again."

There are degrees of severity in both type 1 and type 2 diabetes. Some people need far more insulin than others, depending on their physical muscularity, exercise habits, and diet discipline. My tests were showing that by using the material in this book, I had effectively muscled up and cut back far enough on all sugar and carbs to jump-start my pancreas back into insulin production. Admittedly, this is a rare occurrence. Another person's ability to do the same depends on his or her individual biochemistry and the lifestyle changes he or she is able to make.

My research continued, and I eventually turned up what I was looking for. A physician in Australia, who was studying the effects of nutrition and exercise on both type 1 and type 2 diabetes, was duplicating my discoveries. I uncovered a vast body of information on nutrient deficiencies in type 1 and type 2 diabetes and in supplement regimens recommended by physicians specializing in nutritional therapies in addition to or in place of pharmaceutical therapies. According to Ian E. Brighthope, MD, author of *The Vitamin Cure for Diabetes* (written with Andrew W. Saul, PhD):

> It is claimed that neither type 1 nor type 2 diabetes can be cured. However, I will show in this book that most people who have type 2 diabetes can be cured and come off all or most medications, if they choose to change their lifestyle—eating a healthy diet, beginning a program of regular exercise and taking nutritional supplements. It is far more difficult to reverse type 1 diabetes to this extent, although some people have been able to stop taking their insulin while many, if not most, can reduce their dosage of insulin.

THE RIGHT INFORMATION MAKES ALL THE DIFFERENCE

The reason our nation is so unhealthy is that we are not being given the right information about how to eat and exercise or how to use supplements to our advantage.

I had to go through what I went through to be able to share the positive news that disease is a charging bull, but it can miss us if we step aside with the skill of a matador. Just as I chose to do, you can use the assistance of medical doctors as well as your own resources: diet and exercise. And you can take advantage of a handful of powerful and well-known but underused supplements that Marilyn and I have proved to ourselves are mandatory for growing younger.

This book presents new thinking about how to prevent disease with food, exercise, and supplements. Obviously, the focus is on building you up to greater levels of health than you've ever known before. The correct answers to the questions of what to eat, what supplements to take, and what type of exercise become easy: *whatever will build you up.*

PART ONE

Two Silent Killers

1

Public Enemy Number One: Nutrient Deficiencies

HOW CAN MALNUTRITION RUN RAMPANT IN THE RICHEST NATION ON EARTH?

If you withhold food from someone for several weeks, that person will starve to death. If you give someone just enough nutrition to get by, they won't starve, but some part of them will be dying. In the United States, food is plentiful, but most of it is processed, artificial, and laden with cellular and neurotoxic chemicals, dyes, preservatives, and additives; it is irradiated, fractionated, microwaved, sprayed with pesticides, fungicides, and herbicides; it is stored for long periods or shipped in hot weather; it is contaminated and genetically modified.

Technically, Americans are not starving to death. In fact, we are eating more than enough calories, but we are getting far too few real nutrients. Like a bird attempting to fly with one wing, we're limping along with symptoms that we've been conditioned to expect and accept. If you want more energy but it seems to be slipping away, you're likely deficient in nutrients. The headache or sense of malaise that keeps you from performing at your peak can be traced directly to your diet.

"Paradoxically, Americans are becoming both more obese and more nutrient deficient at the same time. . . . But if all you eat is processed food—and many Americans do—then you will be like the British sailors of the seventeenth century and get scurvy," says Mark Hyman, MD, author of *The Blood Sugar Solution*.

Full-blown malnutrition is an identifiable disease with many names. Some examples, in addition to scurvy, are beriberi, rickets, pellagra, and kwashiorkor. These are not often diagnosed in our country, although doctors should be testing for them in children and adults because one cause of pellagra, for example, is a diet high in corn and low in protein. Those who rely on corn as a staple and eat great quantities of popcorn, chips, and cereals are predisposed to pellagra.

Nutrient deficiencies *are* rampant in our country. "The price the cell pays for being short of micronutrients is DNA damage, which leads to cancer in the future and ages you faster," warns Bruce Ames, PhD, of the University of California, Berkeley. Dr. Ames is a leading voice in the appeal for better health and the prevention of disease through nutritional strategies. Having studied his work and that of many of his colleagues, we are convinced that our country is faced with its own unique malnutrition epidemic, which we call Nutrient Deficiency Disorder (NDD). In the United States, we have enough food to fill our bellies, but our food is nutrient poor, and it is making us sick.

Dr. Ames believes a nutrient-deficient diet plays a role in just about every disease you can name, especially obesity, heart disease, diabetes, cancer, and a vast number of mental disorders. This level of poor nutrition—best described as *just getting by*—is a point along the way to full-blown malnutrition. You are low on the nutrients that you need for optimal health, so you obviously have no chance of being optimally healthy. You're like a tire with a leak—not yet flat, but bumping along in that direction. You're not at the clinical level of duress, but you have many symptoms that indicate that you're not at your highest level of health, either.

You may be suffering from high blood pressure. You may be tired all the time, catching every cold and flu bug that comes along. You may be overweight, underweight, anxious, feeling out of sorts and off balance, or walking around with infections you can't shake. You may be peering into the mirror at wrinkles and gray hair long before you expected them to appear. You may have aches and pains. You may have lost interest in sex because you don't feel well enough or have the energy to enjoy it. You're not clinically sick *yet,* but without a doubt, you're moving in that direction.

When you are in this stage of physical and mental duress, most doctors can't make heads or tails of what's causing your ailments. As long as you have some air in the tire, to them, it's too soon to diagnose a real problem. You receive a patch for the leak. It's some drug that hopefully might stop it. Unfortunately, it most often comes with side effects, which will only cause additional leaks.

Most physicians may be unable to address nutrient deficiencies. The courses they study in medical school amount to a pharmaceutical curriculum. They are trained to fix problems with drugs. If you're eating three or more meals a day, the average medical mind isn't trained to consider malnutrition as a cause of your sickness. Even when a doctor checks your blood, he or she compares the results with bare minimum requirements that actually perpetuate your suffering from Nutrient Deficiency Disorder.

The fact is, the health care system isn't allowing NDD to be diagnosed. Judging from the vending machines and snack tables laden with granola bars and other sweet treats in doctor's offices and hospitals, it's obvious that many of the experts in this system have no clue about the nutrient requirements of your body. They're not even clear about the correct choices of food they themselves need to eat to function at symptom-free levels. You know this is true when you're hospitalized and the food service brings you a tray containing soda and cake and your doctor doesn't even protest.

In a society like ours, seemingly so advanced and blessed with food abundance, there are three areas of health care policy to scrutinize to see why NDD is one of our biggest health problems. These are:

1. Artifacts disguised as food
2. Ridiculous Dietary Reference Intakes
3. Censorship and profits

ARE YOU EATING ARTIFACTS?

In 1940, a very small percentage of our purchased food was processed. Today, that figure is over 90 percent. Processed foods are not foods; they are artifacts, consumed in a society that has been conditioned to accept that industry is the modern mom in the kitchen. Over hundreds of millennia, humans subsisted on natural foods. These can be defined as foods that are growing and alive, or were recently alive, in nature, in the rain and under the sun—all plant foods, meat, eggs, and fish. We ate our food within minutes or hours of gathering it, because there was little opportunity for storage. Even when we no longer hunted and gathered, we still planted our foods in the earth or found them in the rivers, pastures, and meadows where we lived. We could see food's authenticity. This "stuff of life" was what we recognized as food through the generations. Until less than a century ago, there was little possibility of the mass manufacturing, packaging, labeling, warehousing, shipping, and advertising that completely drive what we eat today.

Processed food artifacts include all cereals, sodas, snacks, and breads, as well as canned and packaged foods with long lists of incomprehensible ingredients. Any food made of refined grain and sugar is processed. As are butter substitutes, vegetable oils, and shortenings; deep-fried foods of all kinds; sugared or artificially sweetened soft drinks; all the soy and gluten analogues (including textured vegetable proteins); and all low-fat, animal-free, and fat-free dairy products—especially any protein without fat. This last invention—the low-fat or fat-free food—touted as healthy, wasn't readily available to us before the early 1990s. When it arrived, along with a huge push from the medical community, government agencies, and food manufacturers, obesity rose well past the Centers for Disease Control and

Prevention goal, of being under 15 percent, to 33.8 percent. Obesity has more than doubled since the 1960s.

Protein without fat is an artifact because it's man-made; it is *never* found that way in nature. Protein and fat are sister nutrients occurring in whole foods. Protein completely devoid of fat is an industrialized product. Genetically modified foods are the height of processing. In this case, the industrialization starts at the level of the DNA of the seed that sprouts the food. Other artifacts of this manufactured family dining experience include the junk and fast food served up in plastic and polystyrene cups and dishes, with plastic spoons, forks, and knives.

It's now possible to have complete meals of artifacts throughout life. One-third of all calories in the United States are consumed away from home, and they largely come from processed ingredients and are eaten with processed utensils on processed plates. You have *no idea* what is in your food. And you wonder why your health is plummeting? Most restaurants rely on reheating foods made with the cheapest processed ingredients they can buy. It's all about making food as inexpensive as possible to garner the greatest profits.

The era of artifact eaters is going to astound archaeologists. They will unearth skeletons with missing teeth, malformed arches, distorted spines, bones full of holes, and malformed joints. When they evaluate the waters and streams of this era, they'll wonder at the toxic residues of seemingly tens of thousands of pharmaceutical drugs. They will probably categorize us as *Homo persecutis*—disenfranchised artifact eaters, victims of profit-driven food industries and the most insane of human missteps: when we left the family kitchen to be *convenienced* to death and allowed our food to be industrialized.

Is it true that you can get all the nutrients you need to prevent illness and an early death by eating a balanced diet? How is it possible to eat a balanced diet with a food supply dominated by artifacts? The fact is, the idea of "balanced diet" hardly applies for most of our population. For example, those on a vegan diet (who mistakenly believe that they're on the healthiest path) are eating an unbalanced and highly processed animal-free diet.

Some experts, like Dr. Ames, believe there is an urgent need to revise the DRI (Dietary Reference Intake, the daily intake level of nutrients required for healthy individuals, similar to the RDA, Recommended Dietary Allowance) and emphasize vitamin supplementation in far higher doses. In an article in the April 2002 issue of the *American*

Journal of Clinical Nutrition, Dr. Ames and his colleagues reported that "about 50 human genetic diseases due to defective enzymes can be remedied or ameliorated" through high-dose nutrient therapy, and that therapy can at least partially restore defective enzyme activity.

A team of physicians and researchers known as the Independent Vitamin Safety Review Panel made the following recommendation to the US government: "Government-sponsored nutrient recommendations, such as the US RDA, are not keeping pace with recent progress in nutrition research. . . . The public has been asked to consume far too little of many . . . key nutrients. Inadequate intake, and inadequate standards to judge intake, have resulted in widespread nutrient inadequacy, chronic disease, and an undernourished but overweight population. . . . Raising the RDA/DRI will save lives and improve health. . . . Clinical and subclinical nutrient deficiencies are among the main causes of our society's greatest healthcare problems. Cancer, cardiovascular disease, mental illness, and other diseases are caused or aggravated by poor nutrient intake. The good news is that scientific evidence shows that adequately high consumption of nutrients helps prevent these diseases."

The panel concluded, "In the past, over-conservative government-sponsored standards have encouraged dietary complacency. People have been led to believe that they can get all the nutrients they need from a 'balanced diet' of processed foods. That is not true. For adequate vitamin and mineral intake, a diet of unprocessed, whole foods, along with the intelligent use of nutritional supplements, is more than just a good idea: it is essential."

NDD AND CENSORSHIP

The US National Library of Medicine is the most prestigious archive of scientific findings in the world. It is politically biased and arbitrarily classifies some medical journals as "good" and others as "blacklisted." How does the archive decide what to accept and what to blacklist? We don't know, but the result is that both you and your doctor are deprived of the ability to access decades of peer-reviewed science that can help move you from nutrient deficient to a state of optimal health.

The "good" journals are easy to access on the Internet through an enormous database called MEDLINE, a free service that is provided by the National Library of Medicine and the National Institutes of Health, both supported by your tax dollars. We're not saying this isn't money well spent—unless, that is, you're interested in finding out something about NDD and what doctors have to say about the successful reversal of this underlying cause of disease.

Since the 1920s, leading biochemists have foreseen impending epidemics of disease. The writing was on the laboratory wall. In an effort to prevent the tragedy now bearing down on us, these scientists published remarkable research on nutrients, in the hope that nutrient awareness would filter down to the public. Specifically, Roger Williams, PhD, of the University of Texas, who discovered many of the B-complex vitamins and authored one of the main textbooks on biochemistry used nationwide in medical schools, lamented that medical doctors weren't interested in nutritional therapies. They preferred more heroic measures, such as surgery and drugs. In a personal crusade for prevention, Dr. Williams wrote seven books on nutrition for the mainstream, turning directly to the general population to prevent increasingly widespread suffering. He was not alone. There were dozens of dedicated biochemists also fighting to be heard, but they were muzzled, prevented from a public discussion on proven, inexpensive, and safe nutritional therapies. This idea simply didn't fit the model of the profit-centered pharmaceutical industry. Nonetheless, the dissenters fought on, because they understood that pharmaceuticals were completely foreign to the biochemistry of the human body. On the other hand, the nutrients these biochemists recommended were identical, nontoxic molecules that comprise the very structure of the human body.

Two-time Nobel laureate Linus Pauling, PhD, gave these biochemists and other like-minded medical scientists a field of their own when he coined the term *orthomolecular medicine,* first discussed in *Science* magazine in 1968. He began to compile their decades of work in the *Journal of Orthomolecular Medicine.* Published since then, with authoritative research on nutritional therapies rather than drugs, this journal is "blacklisted" today because of the bias against nutritional solutions in favor of pharmaceutical solutions. Even Dr. Pauling's own research in that journal cannot be included in MEDLINE! (Of course, the issue is profits. Nutrients cannot be patented.) You have no access to Dr. Pauling's research in MEDLINE, nor do medical doctors who turn to that database as a resource, nor do journalists. Even the research for which Dr. Pauling won his first Nobel Prize is excluded! Other valuable, life-saving research papers written by equally prestigious scientists and physicians are missing from MEDLINE, too. These are scientists who have discovered how we could use nutrition and nutrients to prevent and reverse some of today's killer diseases.

One of the repercussions of this repression of decades of peer-reviewed research from scientists, who are experts in the field of nutrition, is that prominent media voices run frequent campaigns of fear against nutrients proved to be indispensable to your body's health. Because of this censorship and misinformation, otherwise reputable journalists take a dim view of nutrients. Yet vitamins have a safety record that is unparalleled in the history of pharmaceuticals. Statistics are available from the American Association of Poison Control Centers' National Poison Data System. The center's 203-page annual report, published in 2011 in the journal *Clinical Toxicology,* shows no deaths from multivitamins, any of the B vitamins, or vitamins A, C, D, or E. On the other hand, if Dr. Ames's contention that more than 50 diseases are caused by nutrient deficiencies is correct, then over the decades, the number of people who have died from nutrient deficiency–related illness could quite possibly reach well into the tens of millions.

You may be a victim of Nutrient Deficiency Disorder. Your neighbor may be a victim. Anyone you know who is stricken with heart disease, cancer, obesity, diabetes, mental illness, or one of so many other common ailments that we are conditioned to accept as natural in the process of aging is likely suffering from NDD. You deserve to know that proven nutritional solutions are available. The FDA, supported by Congress, is continuously fighting to take your supplements away from you, to control any competition that supplements pose to the pharmaceutical companies.

"The drug companies control the passing of laws in their favor," says attorney Jonathan Emord, author of two books that discuss of our health choices, *The Rise of Tyranny* and *Global Censorship of Health Information.* "They write and decide what Congress will pass. They influence the FDA commissioner, push drugs with adverse side effects, and heavily influence the conduct of Congress."

Interviewed by Emord on the Conscious Living blog, Representative Dan Boren of Oklahoma admitted, "There is really no bill that, if the drug industry wants it bad enough, won't get passed."

The campaign is under way, guided by pharmaceutical companies, to "scientifically" discredit the benefits of nutritional supplements, as well as whole foods, in our diet.

CHAPTER 2

Public Enemy Number Two: Sedentary Death Syndrome

OUR ON-THE-COUCH LIFESTYLE IS CAUSING PREMATURE MUSCLE WASTING AND THREATENING OUR LIVES.

Sedentary Death Syndrome, or SeDS, is the term developed by more than 200 leading physiologists to bring attention to the growing epidemic of physical inactivity and poor nutrition and their relationship to chronic, preventable diseases. It is estimated that 60 percent of all Americans are currently at risk for premature disability or death due to poor nutrition and a sedentary lifestyle, and some of them are children.

Approximately 2.5 million Americans will die prematurely in the next 10 years as a result of SeDS; that's greater than the number of deaths related to alcohol, guns, motor vehicles, illicit drug use, and sexual behavior combined. Researchers call SeDS the second-largest threat to public health and expect it to add as much as $3 trillion to health care costs over the next 10 years.

Frank W. Booth, PhD, a professor of biomedical sciences at the University of Missouri-Columbia, warns of this serious health threat and the link between physical inactivity and disease. He cites 35 known serious health conditions that are caused or worsened by physical inactivity, including arrhythmia, arthritis pain, breast cancer, colon cancer, congestive heart failure, depression, gallstone disease, heart attack, hypertension, obesity, osteoporosis, peripheral vascular disease, respiratory problems, sleep apnea, stroke, and type 2 diabetes.

The population in nursing homes will quadruple in the next 50 years, driven, in part, by the premature onset of diseases from sedentary lifestyles. "That bulge, coupled with the spiraling number of obese children, will bankrupt the health care system," Dr. Booth predicts.

A study reported in the *Archives of Internal Medicine* in January 2008 proves that exercise has a powerful impact on extending life span on the cellular level. If you're willing to exercise even moderately, you can reduce genetic aging by as much as 10 years.

Inside the center, or nucleus, of a cell, our genes are located on twisted, double-stranded molecules of DNA called chromosomes. At the ends of the chromosomes are stretches of DNA called telomeres. Picture these telomeres as the plastic tips of the trillions of microscopic shoelaces (chromosomes) that contain your DNA. You've seen what happens when the plastic tip of a shoelace wears off. The lace itself begins to weaken and unravel. Using this image, you can visualize what is happening to your telomeres as you age. Scientists know that the longer your telomeres, the greater your chances for longevity and the slower your body ages.

In the study, British researchers conducted tests on 2,400 sets of twins to measure the length of the telomeres in their DNA, a good indicator of the age potential of DNA. With each cell replication, scientists can see that under normal conditions, telomeres tend to shorten, and as they shorten, the ability of the cell to replicate declines until cell replication is no longer possible. If we can see that telomeres shorten under certain conditions, we can also determine what we need to do to lengthen them. Never before have we had this kind of understanding about how to control our longevity.

The most important finding of the study was the effect of physical activity on the length of telomeres. The researchers concluded that even light activity has a direct effect on lengthening telomeres. This has a powerful impact on extending life span on the cellular level and can reduce genetic aging by as much as 10 years.

Other studies have shown a correlation between physical activity and longevity. One recent report in the *New England Journal of Medicine* suggested that your level of physical fitness is the strongest predictor of your longevity. It studied nearly 17,000 Harvard alumni and determined that "death rates declined steadily as energy expended on such activity [walking, stair climbing, sports] increased." Another large study by researchers at Stanford University and the Veterans Affairs Palo Alto Health Care System, which appeared in the same publication in 2002, showed a similar benefit. In this study, which began in 1987, 6,213 men (average age 59) were given an electrocardiogram (EKG) test while exercising on a treadmill. Before testing, each man also completed a questionnaire about his medical history, current medications, and risk factors for various diseases.

During the exercise test, blood pressure, heart rate, and exercise capacity were monitored, and EKG results were recorded. Based on their medical records and the results of their exercise tests, the men were classified as either having cardiovascular disease or not. Later the researchers reviewed the list of subjects and compared the exercise capacity test results of those men who had died with the results of the men who where still living. It turned out that men with the lowest exercise capacity, according to a follow-up treadmill test, were more than four times more likely to die than men with the highest exercise capacity. This was true regardless of whether the men had cardiovascular disease or not, which implies that exercise may even offset the risks of cardiovascular disease! As exercise capacity increased, the chances of survival increased.

YOU NEED MORE MUSCLE

Sarcopenia (sar-koh-PEEN-ia) is a condition of accelerated muscle wasting that leads to the diseases of premature aging. Identified by the Centers for Disease Control and Prevention (CDC) in 1999, this condition was first considered to be a geriatric disease that became severe in one's seventies. Today, however, muscle wasting can begin in your twenties or even earlier. As you age, your body naturally loses muscle mass at the rate of approximately 1 percent a year after age 30. But when you are sedentary, muscle wasting accelerates, and it can start much earlier in life.

Your very life depends on a healthy ratio of more toned muscle to less fat on your body. Once this healthy ratio is inverted—when you have much more fat than muscle—you expose yourself to the entire chain of the modern killer diseases, including cancer, diabetes, heart attack, obesity, and stroke. If your muscles are wasting, you're in pain. You're also likely to have poor posture, impaired nerve function, and stress on your heart and other organs. Everything in your body is compromised. Blood flow to your abdominal area is obstructed, so digestion is ineffective and you may suffer from constipation, heartburn, indigestion, and irritable bowel syndrome. There is lack of blood flow to the reproductive organs, so you (both men and women) may experience sexual dysfunction, a loss of confidence, and a lack of desire. These conditions of accelerated aging can be traced to sarcopenia caused by a sedentary lifestyle.

Who in their right mind would pursue a life that causes attractive and youthful muscle to disappear from the body, only to be replaced by sagging and flabby fat? Just about everyone in this country, that's who!

Muscle wasting has two deadly side effects. With less muscle, your metabolism slows down. As your metabolism slows, you have less energy to move around. Trapped in inactivity, you gain fat weight, which is inactive flabby tissue, as opposed to active, toned muscle tissue. The less muscle you have, the fewer calories you burn. And, critical to every single symptom of premature aging you're experiencing, the less muscle you have, the less sugar is burned from your blood. The more sugar in your blood, the greater your need for the fat-storing hormone insulin. So muscle wasting not only prevents fat burning but also leads to diabetes and heart and kidney disease.

HIGH BLOOD SUGAR DAMAGES YOUR BRAIN AND MUSCLES

You've heard of diabetic neuropathy—the nerve damage from high blood sugar that can ultimately lead to amputation and death. But this damage to the nerves is only part of the story of high blood sugar, which is directly connected to sarcopenia. Did you know that the nerves in your brain and spinal cord are under siege when your blood sugar is too high? When they are destroyed, and where they are destroyed, the muscles are lost. An early example of this common symptom of nerve damage is the loss of eyesight and hearing. But the greater point we're making is that a lifestyle that causes excess sugar in the blood affects your nerves and, as a result, begins to age you prematurely.

Children are suffering from an unhealthy muscle-to-fat ratio, which in their young bodies is already creating diabetes and obesity. The degree of SeDS in our children, coupled with their diets of processed carbohydrates and sugar, will cause obesity statistics to almost double in 10 years. With slow metabolisms and high blood sugar, our children will be at risk of neuronal damage and compromised brain function. Considering that more than one in six children today are obese, and the majority have an imbalanced muscle-to-fat ratio, the consequences to health care costs will be astronomical. Even the military now recognizes the widespread obesity in children in our country as a threat to our national security. Our obese older teens are being disqualified from military service because they are not strong enough to undergo rigorous training.

Are you suffering from sarcopenia? Do you recall a time in your life when you couldn't eat as much as you did before without gaining weight? Do you remember when you suddenly could no longer fit into jeans you'd been wearing for years? Are you thin but not firm? Are you skinny but soft? Have you noticed that you have less strength? This often happens in your twenties, thirties, or forties, and at this stage, it's the warning sign that you're suffering from early-onset sarcopenia.

When the CDC first identified sarcopenia, it warned us that this condition was already one of the top five health risks in our country. Yet many doctors who advise their patients to lose weight are completely unaware of this disease and of the very real dangers of muscle loss.

The ignorance associated with this epidemic makes muscle wasting a true "silent killer." Worldwide, sarcopenia is not high on the list of concerns. Doctors still think of muscle wasting as a concern only among older populations. *Sarcopenia* isn't a word that's commonly in use in the medical vocabulary, nor are doctors aware that this silent epidemic is causing the obesity that is striking people at every age. You'll rarely hear the word on television talk shows or read it in the newspaper. What is worse is that many people, doctors included, do not recognize that sarcopenia is a major underlying cause of obesity, diabetes, and heart disease, as well as a contributor to arthritis, impotency, osteoporosis, Parkinson's disease, and the loss of eyesight and hearing.

Our goal is to help you realize the danger of a sedentary lifestyle. We want you to experience the very real healing in the body that comes from muscle toning, as opposed to muscle wasting. Visit a nursing home and you will see the end result of sarcopenia in the stooped, bony residents who need assistance to dress, use the bathroom, and move from one place to another. This situation *can* be prevented, starting at any age. If you're groaning as you stand up from a sofa or when you get out of your car, you are already in the clutches of sarcopenia.

For those with eyes to see, Americans at all ages are suffering from skinny-fat (that is, thin but with fat instead of lean skeletal muscle) or corpulent bodies. This is the visible indication of the nationwide loss of the healthy balance between muscle and fat. Practically our entire nation quietly suffers from rampant accelerated muscle wasting, at great cost to our health, our productivity, and our health care budget, and we're totally ignorant of this harmful condition.

Muscle wasting affects everyone. This naturally occurring condition, which most doctors believe begins after age 75, in our opinion begins the day you toss the TV remote control to your toddler instead of putting him on a tricycle. It starts the moment you offer your baby a bottle of fructose-sweetened juice or soda instead of a glass of milk. But we can start to change this dangerous American affliction, and you have already begun to by picking up this book.

PART TWO

How to Prevent NDD and SeDS

CHAPTER **3**

Grow Younger

LEARN HOW TO KEEP YOUR MUSCLES
BUILDING UP RATHER THAN BREAKING DOWN.

Revolutions tend to bring new terms. For example, the earlier book *Fit for Life* introduced *food combining* and *high-water-content food*. To be Young for Life and in good shape and good health, you have to be *anabolic*. On the other hand, if you're aging too fast, you are becoming *catabolic*. It is important to understand these two words—*anabolic* and *catabolic*—if you want to get a grip on your health.

Anabolism is the process of building and repairing strong cells. This word describes a key process of how your body keeps you alive and well.

Catabolism is a two-phase process. Phase one is the healthy one during which your body tears down old cells that are ready to be replaced. However, a second, unwelcome phase of catabolism occurs when your body can't find the building blocks it requires to start the anabolic (rebuilding) process. Since those building blocks must come from protein, your body is forced to tear down your precious protein-rich muscle tissue. This happens when you are nutrient deficient. Without the proper amount of protein in your diet, your body will actually cannibalize its own muscle to accomplish cell repair. This tearing down of your muscle tissue also contributes to sarcopenia, the muscle wasting we learned about in Chapter 2. This is why you want to do what it takes to keep yourself out of this phase of catabolism.

Your body is smart. It has the intelligence to preserve your brain, heart, and other vital organs for as long as it can. But since most of your tissue is built from protein (the exception being your brain, which is 60 percent fat), to repair these vital tissues and keep them running, your body will automatically tear down your precious and hard-earned muscle tissue for the amino acids it needs to support and preserve your vital organs. When you've pushed this deprivation too far and your body has no more muscle to turn to, it will begin to forgo "less important" repairs, and an organ is going to fail you. Since your heart is a muscle, a serious end point of excessive catabolism is the thinning out of your heart muscle.

Look at this in simple terms. Your body is a house that needs repairing. But before you can even arrange for the delivery of construction materials, the house is already falling down around you. This is what happens when catabolism outstrips anabolism in the process of building new cells. It's a very slight tip of the scale, but it's one you want to prevent at all costs. You want to be building strong, youthful cells with an abundance of construction materials available. The alternative—to put it in blunt terms—is a whole lot of pain and suffering.

Anabolism and catabolism are the two most important phases of your metabolism. Your metabolism is the summation of all the molecular processes that occur within you to keep you alive. Metabolism is commonly measured in pace. People who have a "fast metabolism" usually can eat whatever they want and not gain weight. Those who have a "slow metabolism" typically gain weight easily.

When you leave home on your way to work or to drive the kids to school and all you've had is coffee, you're rushing headlong into catabolism. When you skip a meal or grab something quick and processed in the grain or sugar family that your body can't immediately identify as the building blocks it needs, you ignore your body's need for protein and force it to search for those proteins in your muscles. Your body doesn't wait for the proper nutrients to come along; its repair work is going on constantly.

The Young for Life program is about maintaining life at the highest level. Focusing on keeping your body in an anabolic state is the most constructive choice you can make. Engineers know that it takes more work to build a structure than it does to demolish one. Have you ever watched a wrecking ball take down an entire building in just a few days? Construction of that building may have taken months, even years. In the same way, it's far easier to break down precious muscle than to build it up. The constructive nature of anabolism requires your attention. It's worth giving it your attention! Your body puts in more effort for anabolism, and this means it burns more calories in the process, helping you shed excess fat and become fitter and younger looking.

In research recently reported in the *American Journal of Epidemiology*, Americans were studied for 14 years to determine the effect that being sedentary had on life span. Past research has linked a sedentary lifestyle to degenerative diseases, such as type 2 diabetes, obesity, and heart disease, but not to total mortality. The report showed that people who sat around for more than 6 hours a day and exercised little had a much higher mortality risk—94 percent higher for women and 48 percent higher for men. This is an example of the danger zone of catabolism.

Your body is forced to consume its muscle when there is a protein deficiency in your diet. Your muscle will also deteriorate if you fail to stay active enough to stimulate growth and maintenance. These two factors are extremely common in our carbohydrate-obsessed, processed

Live a Strong (and Long) Life

Strength training is longevity training. In research published in the *British Medical Journal*, now called *BMJ*, scientists analyzing dozens of studies on longevity found that men who could lift more weight with their legs and arms tended to live longer. The group found that muscle power protects against falls and fractures, osteoporosis, and other diseases associated with aging, especially against cancer. According to the researchers, the analysis suggests that "it might be possible to reduce all cause[s of] mortality among men by promoting regular resistance training involving the major muscle groups of the upper and lower body, two or three days a week."

food–focused, sedentary culture. Anytime there is a shortage of protein and other vital nutrients, your body interprets this as a downward spiral toward starvation and goes directly into the metabolic reactions associated with stress. Your stressed-out brain sends the age-old emergency alarm to your body to hold on to your fat in order to avoid the starvation that it perceives on the horizon.

Since the dawn of human existence, this signal has caused muscle breakdown and fat storage. According to the latest data from the National Health and Nutrition Examination Survey of 2007–08, the number of obese American adults exceeds the number of those who are merely overweight. More than 35 percent of Americans are obese, compared with more than 33 percent who are overweight. Add these together and you have nearly 70 percent of Americans at serious risk of catabolism. This is an alarming and accelerating crisis of muscle loss and fat storage.

Add the skinny-fat population to this group. These are underweight people who are soft, flabby, and lacking muscle tone. They, like the overweight and obese, are in a state of muscle loss and fat storage. Now we're closing in on nearly our *entire* population in the crisis of catabolism. This is not just a physical problem. When you fail to exercise properly and to eat the nutritious foods required for anabolism and more youthful cells, instead forcing your body to break down muscle for nutrients, you struggle with feelings of stress, depression, unclear thinking, and irritability, as well as with the inability to solve problems or reason effectively.

ENTER THE ANABOLIC ZONE

Anabolism is your ideal state, but you have to earn it through the right food and exercise choices. *You* are the most important player in this process. It's up to you to give your body what it requires to build the youngest, strongest, and healthiest cells. As you support your body's anabolic process with the right nutrition and the right exercise, you'll see and feel the results, including:

- A trimmer belly
- Muscles that are firm rather than soft, flat, or stringy
- Glowing and more youthful skin
- Naturally stronger nails
- A smaller waist and flatter, toned abs
- Lifted breasts and a chest that's less saggy
- Trimmer and stronger legs with more sexy definition
- Better posture
- Shapely arms and shoulders
- Boosted brain power and creativity
- Optimism and a more upbeat attitude
- An end to cravings, such as for sugary or salty carb snacks
- Greater energy
- A calmer, more balanced disposition

Anabolism is the secret to staying energized with the proper muscle-to-fat ratio. Anabolism is the key to staying young and the antidote to growing old too fast. It's the next step—a brand-new guiding principle for fighting Nutrient Deficiency Disorder and Sedentary Death Syndrome, which cause disease and decline.

CHAPTER 4

The Surprising Effect of Anabolism on Your Hormones

MANAGING STRESS IS CRUCIAL TO PREVENTING SKINNY-FAT SYNDROME.

Testosterone is the hormone that most helps to promote protein synthesis (muscle tone and shape), strength, youthfulness, higher energy levels, and fat burning. Although testosterone is known as the "male hormone," women have some, too, and it influences those same areas. Women produce testosterone in their adrenal glands and ovaries, men in their adrenal glands and testes. But both men and women can encourage their bodies to release more of this useful hormone by working their muscles with resistance exercises.

In Chapter 29, you will find a 12-minute at-home workout called the Isotonics Routine. The exercises in the program will work the large muscle groups of your body without weights, specifically, your glutes, thighs, back, chest, and shoulders. While doing this routine, you will release testosterone, which means you will be toning muscle through anabolism. As you progress, you will want to make the activities more challenging by adding more sets or by using weights, and you won't even have to think about this. As your body becomes increasingly anabolic, it will naturally lead you to wish for more weight, which means the older you get, the stronger and more youthful you can become.

Now you have the keys to the kingdom. When you use anabolic exercise to release testosterone, you are turning on the hormones that help you slow down and even reverse aging. But this is just the beginning. In this anabolic system, you are influencing several other major hormones, with both your focused techniques and your anabolic food choices. More on those later.

THE DESTRUCTIVE HORMONE

One hormone that you definitely want to manage in your body is cortisol. You may not be familiar with the term, but you know what it is. Often when you're irritable, grouchy, overstressed, or aggressive, cortisol is in control of you. If you wake up in a bad mood, your body could be flooded with cortisol, and you don't even know it. Eating an anabolic food such as plain, unsweetened yogurt will quickly reduce cortisol production. Sugar will also do this, temporarily, for 20 to 30 minutes, but your mood may be far worse after that as sugar plunges you more deeply into cortisol.

Cortisol plays a causal role in sarcopenia. It's the primary catabolic hormone that signals the destruction of your youthful lean muscle

DR. ROCK REPORTS...

Anabolic exercise has been my lifelong sport. I not only use it to shape my body, but I rely on it to stimulate hormonal activity to keep young.

How often do you engage in some form of exercise, thinking, "Ah, I'll work on turning on my libido, and I'll get rid of some wrinkles while I'm doing it"? Never. But that's exactly what you are doing biochemically when you engage in anabolic exercise. Testosterone is proven to be the number one hormone in both sexes for toning muscles. I can vouch for this personally. I'm stronger now in my late fifties than I was in my thirties. Testosterone is also the hormone in both sexes for sexual arousal, desire, and stimulation. I can vouch for those effects of anabolic exercise as well!

tissue (as well as your positive attitude) while telling your body to store fat. To fight cortisol, you need to perform anabolic exercises like those in the Isometrics Workout found in Chapter 6 and eat anabolic foods before and immediately after exercising. We will show you how important it is to eat anabolic meals three to four times a day, with few exceptions.

As indicated, cortisol also triggers irritability, which should be an immediate alert to you to do something anabolic with nutrition, to reduce your cortisol level and stop its activity. Left unchecked, the stress causes fight-or-flight behavior that can be borderline aggressive as your body literally begins to break itself down. What follows logically is the urgency for fat storage as the brain receives the signal of the first stages of starvation and preserves fuel for the heart and other organs. In Part 3, we'll show you exactly how to remedy fight-or-flight with proper nutrition.

Cortisol is one of the primary steroids secreted by the adrenal glands. An excess of this hormone not only causes fat storage, but also can trigger osteoporosis. In fact, medical doctors are reluctant to prescribe corticosteroids precisely because they can cause severe bone loss. Cortisol not only breaks down muscle; it also weakens bones!

Interestingly, too much cardio exercise, or too much of any physical activity to the point of exhaustion, can trigger your body to release this stress hormone. But a long, stressful meeting in a boardroom will also stimulate cortisol production, especially if all you had to eat was coffee and doughnuts. To control this hormone, it is critical to eat regularly— not to skip meals or grab a muffin and coffee on the run, but to eat good, nutritious food.

Insulin is the fat-storing hormone, and glucagon is the fat-burning hormone. These two hormones compete directly with each other for control of your shape. When your insulin spikes too high—which always happens after eating the simple sugars in sweets, sodas, white flour and other refined grains, and potatoes—glucagon and the fat-burning mechanisms it releases are automatically turned off.

Glucagon is also produced in the pancreas, but like the Red Sox and the Yankees, insulin and glucagon fight. Bodybuilders who can't have one shred of fat covering their hard-earned muscles during competition know how to manage insulin, to keep glucagon turned on. You can learn to do this, too—without becoming muscle-bound—simply by controlling your insulin and glucagon production through the foods you choose to eat.

YOUR YOUTH HORMONES

There are two hormones you must go out of your way to increase to stimulate antiaging: human growth hormone (HGH) and insulin-like growth factor (IGF), which work in concert. IGF is one of the few substances that will actually create new muscle stem cells in your body. This is the finest form of anabolism. You can actually add new muscle tissue to compensate for the loss of muscle tissue from sarcopenia. We have directly and dramatically experienced the phenomenon of how anabolic exercise stimulates the production of this hormone team to create the foundation for a younger body and mind. The reason you age and lose muscle mass is because your body releases less and less IGF as the decades pass, and your body isn't using insulin to stop the breakdown of your muscles overnight the way it used to. The secret to continuing the release of quantities of IGF is to challenge your body with progressive resistance training and to supplement that with certain peptide nutrients at the right times of day.

Peptide nutrients are the wave of the future, and one that has already been used effectively for decades is arginine, a protein nutrient that releases growth hormone when taken on an empty stomach in the

Muscle Up to Prevent Diabetes

According to a recent study in the *Journal of Clinical Endocrinology & Metabolism,* the proportion of muscle mass on the body, built with progressive resistance training, may lower the risk of type 2 diabetes. For each 10 percent increase in the ratio of muscle mass to total body weight, researchers found an 11 percent reduction in insulin resistance and a 12 percent reduction in prediabetes.

morning, before your workout. Although there is currently no DRI for arginine, we like to take 3 to 6 grams. If you want to try that, too, that's good—but start on the low end. There is an abundance of research documenting arginine's safety and efficacy, as well as its potential side effects. Check with your doctor before trying arginine, especially if you have heart problems or asthma, are pregnant, or are taking other medications (but you already knew that).

Having more IGF in your body also raises your libido. It prevents wrinkling, signals fat burning, and triggers deeper sleep. You could spend as much as $36,000 a year for medically supervised injections of HGH to trigger IGF. We don't advise that. We want you to make your own. Realize that HGH is a natural substance. We will teach you the secret technology of progressive resistance training that will help you produce these important hormones naturally. Brick by brick, a house is made; you don't do it in one day. In the next chapter, we'll introduce simple isometric exercises to get you started. It's one that you can do anywhere. Be willing to master this 60-second foundation of anabolism and it will naturally take you as far as you can go. Fitting into jeans you never thought you could wear again is worth the effort alone. But you will also enjoy the admiration of others who will recognize in you new energy, lightheartedness, and joy. We guarantee that those who know you will see and hear the difference in you; they will remark that you seem to get younger each year.

CHAPTER **5**

Isometrics
THE NO-EXCUSES, NO-FRILLS, EASIEST FORM OF ANABOLIC EXERCISE

We are going to make a bold declaration: With just 60 to 90 seconds of exercise every day, you can firm your chest, lift your breasts, tighten and flatten your waist, sculpt gorgeous, toned arms and shoulders, and create rock-hard buns. Of course, if you spend even more time— say, 5 minutes—and use this routine more frequently during the day, you'll gain those results far more quickly. But it's true: You can experience the taut feeling of stronger, well-toned muscles with just seconds of exercise a day. Best of all, you will have escaped the clutches of muscle wasting. And this program is easy. It can be done sitting, standing, or even lying down.

Isometrics has long been shown to be an incredibly effective option for strengthening and shaping muscle. Our nation lost this uniquely safe and gimmick-free approach to toning muscles as the fitness industry raced to create special exercise machines and toning devices and promoted competitions, exhibitions, and countless aerobic exercises. The business of fitness is obsessed with finding the next new thing, overcomplicating something that should be quite natural. As a result, many people fell out of their natural tendency for physical activity. *Exercise* became a bad word for far too many people who became turned off. Exercise was now too demanding, too difficult, and too expensive. It required outfitting and training, and it was just too intimidating. At a most desperate time in our history, when our population is far too out of shape, isometrics is one of the easiest, most affordable, and fastest ways to put an end to flab, excess weight, and skinny-fat obesity.

An isometric exercise requires no equipment. It relies simply on the maximum contraction of a muscle. Your muscle is toned without movement, remaining in a fixed position. When you use isometrics, your muscle cells release insulin-like growth factor (IGF), but this hormone could just as well be named *intrinsic tone factor,* since that's the effect you'll gain from stimulating its release. For your muscles to tone properly, they must contract fully. This is why isometric exercise is so effective. Even a brief 6-second isometric hold of a muscle, once a day, every day, will build a stronger body that sidesteps sarcopenia.

HOW FROGS CONTRIBUTE TO ENDING FLABBY MUSCLES

The basic principle of isometric exercise was discovered in the 1920s. Scientists noticed that when one leg of a frog was tied down over a period of time, it grew significantly stronger than the leg left free. This is because when the frog tried to move the bound leg, it had to activate more muscle fibers. (No one knows exactly *why* these guys tied down a frog's leg.)

It was not until 1953, however, that two German doctors, Theodor Hettinger and Erich Mueller, at the Max Planck Institute of Molecular Physiology in Dortmund, worked out the implications of this observation and applied them to the human body. They found that while traditional exercise, known as *isotonics*, tones a muscle by moving it, isometrics tones the muscle through a sustained muscle contraction. When you contract or squeeze your glutes, you force them into a tight, fixed position that will soon become their natural shape.

You'll see what we mean if you try this right now, while you're sitting and reading this book: Inhale deeply. Place your right hand on your right thigh, and then press your right foot solidly down against the floor while exhaling. You can feel all the muscles of the leg contracting. Use only about 50 percent of your strength for this warmup contraction. Then, inhale again, and while slowly exhaling and hissing for 6 seconds (more on this in a bit), really press and tense to the maximum. You should feel a subtle pump in the muscles of your leg. You've just begun to tone your legs with a powerful maximum muscle contraction.

Through this immobile contraction, nearly 100 percent of the muscles' thousands of hairlike fibers are stimulated, helping to make you stronger and shapelier. In fact, studies done at the Max Planck Institute showed that those who used isometrics revealed strength gains of at least 300 percent over the other test groups who engaged in *any* other type of exercise. As you tense, you're not moving, but you can feel the muscle hardening. The muscle doesn't shorten or stretch; it firms and remains the same length. This is how you exercise effectively without moving a muscle.

After extensive work with over 5,000 volunteers, Dr. Mueller claimed that a muscle held in an isometric contraction for 6 seconds a day would increase in strength at a rate of over 5 percent a week! In other words, if you tense your glutes as hard as you can for 6 seconds a day, in 15 weeks they will be twice as strong as they are today. If you are willing to spend

6 seconds a day for 1 muscle group, or 60 seconds a day for 10 muscle groups, using this technique for muscle toning can make you immune to our greatest new risk factor for mortality: Sedentary Death Syndrome.

Do you have 60 seconds? Can you spare 6? All we're asking is that you make the life choice to give yourself 6 seconds every waking hour to tone your body. Tone one muscle every hour. Start with your neck, then work your chest, arms, abs, glutes, legs—you get the idea. Now, you may be wondering . . .

In your body, you have both involuntary and voluntary muscles. Your heart is an example of an involuntary muscle. It continues to pump around the clock because your survival depends on it. The biceps muscle of your upper arm is a voluntary muscle. It tenses only when it is called upon to do so.

Isometric exercise can benefit all of the 600-plus voluntary muscles in your body. Even though you have billions of muscle fibers, if you are the typical sedentary American, you use only a tiny fraction of these fibers. If, for example, you use your biceps muscle to pick up a cup of coffee or a beer, hardly any of the potential of the muscle fibers is activated. When you brush your hair, you use only a few fibers of the biceps muscle. But if you lift a baby, you will fire more of the biceps by necessity. If you lift a heavy piece of equipment, you will fire even more. Now suppose the only activity you gave your biceps was combing your hair or bringing a can of soda or cup of coffee to your lips. Only the few fibers involved would be toned, and the rest would be flabby. Because most Americans rarely use their muscles, the majority of their muscle fibers are flabby from lack of use.

Isometric exercises are relevant for men, women, and children. Everyone has the same muscles. The same exercises that develop a woman's legs will develop a man's legs. The same exercise that develops a man's chest will help shape and lift a woman's cleavage. The exercises that tighten the abs or the buns are the same for both sexes. When children learn isometrics—and they should—they learn early in life how to take control of the strength of their muscles with simple, natural methods.

This is a personal approach to anabolism that is always at your command. You can do 1 isometric for 6 seconds every hour, or you may choose to do 10 in about a minute. You may choose to begin at home when you wake up, and then repeat these exercises at work, or in the afternoon or evening. If you choose to contract a muscle more than once, you are giving yourself a bonus. *You* are in control. The main thing is that you suit your own schedule and inclinations. But whatever you choose, please *do* choose to start using isometrics to improve or regain your health. In exercise, as in everything in life, the greatest power you have is the power of choice.

THREE PRINCIPLES OF ISOMETRICS

1. Deep Breathing Burns Fat.

Too often we forget to breathe, or we use only the uppermost part of our lungs for breathing. Fat burning or combustion requires oxygen, so the more deeply you breathe, the more fat you burn. The late Jack LaLanne is reported to have said, "The harder you breathe, the more oxygen you take into your bloodstream and the faster you burn off fat. It's very similar to your fireplace; the more air you give the fire, the faster it burns."

Philip Rice, MD, who has worked his whole life with delinquent children, says 55 percent of delinquency in minors is caused by oxygen starvation. Unfortunately, the overweight people of our nation suffer from oxygen starvation. It is up to you to deliver the oxygen to your cells to combust the fats they are holding. You may have been a sitter or shallow breather up until now, but we're going to help you combat that with an easy isometric exercise to immediately become more physically active.

Here is a special technique for ensuring that you breathe properly: Exhale so that you make an audible hissing sound, *S-S-S-S,* with your teeth *almost* clenched together. Try it. Before you make the hissing exhalation, be certain that you have inhaled deeply. You can make the exhalation silently, or you can use the audible hiss: *S-S-S-S.* In martial arts the custom is to use the audible hiss, which is known to focus the mind on the action, tighten the body, and build internal strength. If you are in an elevator going to work, standing with a bunch of office workers, use the silent hiss. You don't want to *hiss* anyone off!

You can become stronger, healthier, and happier just by learning to breathe more deeply. When you practice your isometric exercise, use the following steps to incorporate fat-burning breathing:

Step 1: Inhale deeply before you contract a muscle.

Step 2: Exhale for 6 seconds, "one-one thousand," and so on, making the *S-S-S-S* sound as you begin the warmup contraction, exerting only about 50 percent of your strength. This is for safety, to condition your muscle and prepare it for the maximum exertion. (We haven't actually gotten to the muscles yet; this is just the breathing exercise, which is so important that you'll definitely want to practice it.)

Step 3: Inhale deeply again.

Step 4: Exhale for 6 seconds while hissing, exerting greater than 50 percent and up to 100 percent if you can do it.

As you breathe and learn this system, you'll be practicing a powerful but long-overlooked exercise principle that doesn't require any equipment. To apply this principle at the gym, inhale deeply before you move a weight, then exhale slowly as you move it. Continue inhalations and exhalations throughout your repetitions.

2. Mental Focus Brings *Results.*

The physiological truth is, if your mind isn't focused on the muscle you're working, the muscle will not respond as effectively. Take the headphones off during your routine if it's your desire to put 100 percent of your mental focus on the muscle you're working. One hundred percent effort, plus focus, equals 100 percent results. *Think* that muscle into sexy shapeliness! Partial focus, no matter how great the effort, yields partial results.

You may argue, "Well, I do better when I have music blasting in my ears as I work out." We all love music, and it is fine on the treadmill, but when sculpting your body, you need *total* focus.

If you are willing to give this system your all, you'll feel and see the results we're promising practically from the moment you start. You can use isometrics anywhere, and you can benefit from just minutes a day of focused concentration. The exercises require no equipment, and in most cases, *nobody even knows you're doing them.*

3. Prioritize Your Weak Areas.

The key to success is to first work on the body part that nags you the most. If you're working your arms, but you notice that it's the backs of your arms, or triceps, that are the flabbiest, tone them first. If you're working your legs, and it's the inner thigh you're most concerned about, work that first. If you're yearning for tighter abdominals, work them first.

Keep in mind that you are not required to move a muscle. You are only contracting the muscle. With this technique, you push with force against an immovable resistance: the back of your chair or an opposing muscle group, for example. You might push bent arms back to tone your triceps. You might put your left hand against your right hand in front of you to build your chest muscles. If you are already working with weights, you can use this principle and simply hold the weight and contract the muscle fully at the top, middle, or bottom of your movement.

Who Has Time to Exercise? *You* do! We've worked it out for you. We've provided a shortcut that will help you get back in the game. The technique of isometric exercise is completely natural to your body's needs and completely user-friendly. You and you alone know when you're contracting a muscle to its max. While you're sitting in your desk chair or your children are playing around you, you can be toning your muscles. While you're watching TV, do a few minutes of isometrics during the commercials.

Will Isometrics Bulk Me Up? No! It's going to sculpt you! Many women avoid resistance exercise because they fear they will become muscular and bulky. They shouldn't worry. Only heavy weightlifting creates Incredible Hulk muscles. You already have plenty of muscle, although you may not be able to see it right now. It's already there, hidden beneath a layer of fat. Isometrics is a unique method of bringing out your sexy shapeliness. As the muscle tones, it burns off the fat that is covering it, little by little. Your muscles will emerge nicely toned. You may even increase your muscle mass, but you won't have muscles bulging through your T-shirt. Isometric exercises are for toning, not bulking. Do the exercises outlined in the next chapter and you will quickly see how they will make you more athletic and graceful. Your greater muscle tone will provide the stability and strength to move through life with more power and confidence.

CHAPTER **6**

The Isometrics Workout

HEAD-TO-TOE FITNESS IN JUST 60 SECONDS

T his no-excuse, no-frills shaping workout will take you only 60 seconds. Read through the whole routine, or just work your way down the list, learning one exercise at a time. These exercises are easy to learn and remember because you're working your body from head to toe in a logical sequence. This is not random movement, but precise stimulation of a targeted muscle through a 6-second contraction. You can use these exercises one or two at a time, or you can use the entire routine as often as you'd like during the day. Most important to remember is the 50-percent warm-up contraction, especially in the beginning. You must signal to your muscle that you're about to tone it before the maximum contraction.

1. SMILE

Your face contains about 17 of the most important appearance muscles. Let's make your face more youthful by exercising all of them. There is nothing more appealing than a big smile. And it's practical—a mechanical tool to help you enjoy your life and whatever you're doing. Without being aware of it, you may actually be exercising your frown muscles! Even if you are happy on the inside, your face may be frozen in a frown because you've overused those muscles.

How to do it:

• Inhale. As you exhale and hiss, smile as wide as you can and really feel the tension in your facial muscles. As you relax, you will notice that you will naturally carry more of a smile throughout the day. This exercise brings immediate benefit as other people return your smile.

2. ADIOS, PAIN IN THE NECK

Neck pain can be caused by weak upper back and neck (trapezius) muscles, and it's easy to fix.

How to do it:

• Lift your shoulders up toward your ears as you inhale deeply. Tighten and squeeze until they tremble, and then hiss as you release. Don't do this with your shoulders back or forward, but in the normal position of good posture. Do this often to bring plenty of blood into these muscles; the weakness and inflammation that are causing this problem should disappear.

3. GET A GRIP

This move works all the muscle fibers in the upper back and shoulders.

How to do it:

• Sit up straight in a chair. Inhale deeply. Reach down and grip the seat. Try your best to lift it while still sitting in it. Exhale slowly for 6 seconds while making the hissing sound, or silently, if need be, as you pull up on the seat 50 percent. Put your mind into the contraction and make those 6 seconds count by lifting with half your force. Repeat the process with an inhalation, and on your second repetition, lift to the maximum if you feel ready; if not, the 50 percent will benefit you well. Let your arms and shoulders tremble as you lift harder while counting to 6 and hissing. You just worked your upper back and shoulders. You just made the muscle fibers stronger.

4. SHAPELY SHOULDERS

Shapely shoulders on women are sexy. On men, well-toned shoulders are masculine. Increased strength in your shoulders will bring you benefits in any sport you play, including tennis, golf, and swimming. With stronger shoulders, you can easily pick up your children or grandchildren, or your groceries. Strong shoulders will benefit you in a hundred ways, from lifting objects to simply looking better.

Your shoulder muscles (deltoids) are made up of three sections: the front, side, and rear. The effect is quite amazing even if you develop just the side delt and rear delt, and it couldn't be easier. As you add a little shape to the side delt, your waist actually appears more slender, and so does your arm. For a more chiseled look, do the following exercises as you sit at your desk.

How to do it:

• Side delt. Place your forearms firmly against the inside arms of your desk chair and push out. Inhale deeply. Hiss as you exhale for 6 seconds.

Use only 50 percent of your strength the first time. Now repeat with maximum isometric contraction of the muscle if you are ready.

• Rear delt. Sit in your chair and inhale deeply. Bend one arm and push it against the back of the chair, as if you were planning to elbow someone behind you. Now, as you exhale and hiss, keep your upper arm fully pressed against the back of the chair as if you were trying to push it away from you. Repeat with the other arm. This is an isometric exercise, so no swinging or punching!

5. THE CHEST QUEST

Both men and women desire a perfectly developed chest as part of their total-body transformation. Women can actually add lift to their breasts by toning their chest and back muscles. You'll even be comfortable in fitted dresses without wearing a bra. It's totally possible!

A well-developed chest is a sign of strength and vitality, indicating a healthy pair of lungs and a healthy heart. It's not the size of the chest that attracts attention—for women or for men—so much as the ability to hold the breasts or chest up. Building the pectorals will reduce sag and create lift, and it can add an inch or two of measurement as well. In addition, the larger the chest and breasts in both men and women, the smaller the waist appears. The focus is symmetry and a balanced body. It's the magic of body sculpting.

Let's start building your chest/breasts from the bottom up. Your chest muscle has five parts: lower, middle, upper, inner (cleavage), and outer. Each is easy to work with just one isometric exercise and variations. The outer chest is stimulated by most of these movements, so no separate exercise is necessary.

How to do it:

• Lower. Stand straight and tall, place your palms together, clasping your hands, but do not interlock the fingers. Let your hands meet below your navel. Inhale deeply, and then push one hand against the other and resist. As in all of these exercises, use 50 percent of your maximum effort on the warmup. On the second repetition, use your full power. Concentrate and push as hard as you can, and when you think you are pushing as hard as you can, push even harder. Remember to exhale for 6 seconds and hiss. Put your mind into your chest muscle for 6 seconds. You want to make the most of this short exercise session. This exercise, done with focus and intensity, will definitely build the lower chest muscles.

• **Middle.** Bring your hands up to the center of your chest. Inhale and do your warmup isometric (or iso, for short), clasping your hands and pressing them together. Now inhale again. Tense your chest, begin your exhalation, and push for 6 seconds, hissing and pushing as hard as you possibly can. Your hands should shake. You can *hiss* your flat, sagging chest goodbye.

• **Upper.** Bring your hands up to forehead level and clasp them together. Inhale. Exhale and hiss as you warm up. Inhale again, and then press your hands together hard, hard, harder! Tense your chest muscles and hiss for 6 seconds as your hands shake with effort. Feel that oxygen? Feel that deep breathing? Oxygen burns fat. You're getting rid of stale air, oxygenating your body and brain, burning fat, and clearing your head to feel more alive. This beats antidepressant pills, which will definitely not develop your chest.

• **Inner (cleavage).** Bring your forearms together in front of your chest, as if holding your hands in prayer. Your elbows should be pressed together and raised so that your upper arms are parallel to the floor; hands in prayer are just above eye level. Inhale deeply. Exhale and do the warmup, pressing and resisting at 50 percent of full effort. Inhale again. Press your forearms against each other with as much force as you can generate, until you shake. Now intensify the pressure as you exhale and hiss. This will help to bring in the center cut of your chest. Focus! And really tense your chest muscles, not your arms. Now go turn some heads!

6. GORGEOUS "GUNS"

The biceps brachii on the upper and front part of your arm is probably the best-known muscle. It's the one kids flex when you ask them to show you their muscles. This is such an easy muscle to work, and you can do it sitting down. To fight the flabby, saggy "bat wings" on the backs of the arms that women detest, work your triceps, the muscles directly opposite your biceps. There's an easy move for that, too.

How to do it:
• **Beautiful biceps.** Make fists with both hands. Bend your right arm in front of you at a 90-degree angle and keep your right elbow tucked

into your rib cage. Cross your left fist over your right arm just below your wrist. Inhale. Put your mind into your muscle and slowly pull your right arm upward while resisting downward with your left fist at 50 percent maximum effort for the warmup. Inhale and repeat, pulling and resisting until you feel your arm trembling, counting to 6 as you exhale and hiss. You should feel tension in the back of your left arm—your triceps brachii muscle is working, which is a bonus. Switch arms and repeat.

• Taut triceps. While standing, make a fist with your right hand and position it upright, as if you were holding a bottle. Place your fist firmly in the palm of your left hand so that both hands are approximately 3 inches below belt level. Your arms should be slightly bent at a 120-degree angle. (At 90 degrees your arm would be bent at a right angle, parallel to the floor. At 180 degrees it would be perpendicular to the floor, hanging at your side. You're holding it in the middle of those positions.) Inhale and press your fist down into the open palm of your left hand, using 50 percent of your power. As you exhale, hiss and resist. Inhale again and repeat at maximum effort, keeping your focus on how taut you are making your triceps. The more you work the triceps in this fashion, the faster the results. Switch arms and repeat.

7. BLUE RIBBON ABS

Why do we place such value on firm, tight abs? The explanation can be traced far back into distant history. It started with yoga, the original foundation for the martial arts. Specifically, a Buddhist yogi, Bodhidharma, left Kolkata around AD 500 and traveled over the rugged and dangerous mountains of Tibet to enter China. The journey through the wilds was perilous. This powerful person became the sixth Buddha, the first patriarch of the Zen Buddhist lineage.

As he began teaching Buddhism, villagers started to bring gold and other valuables to the temple. The gold and valuables attracted thieves, so Bodhidharma taught the priests what is known as a "hard style" in the philosophy of martial arts—the anabolic martial art of kung fu. He also taught the villagers a form of "soft style," which evolved into tai chi. Hard style was *only* for the monks, so that they could protect the temples, because the beauty and wealth of the temple was the "bank" of the village. Hard style toughened the monks and developed in them the powers of offense and defense. Soft style helped the villagers develop flexibility and peace of mind.

Among the exercises Bodhidharma taught the monks were isometrics to develop a firm midsection so that they could absorb punishment during combat without injury. According to Bodhidharma, the midsection held the source of human power or "qi" (chi). For the kung fu masters, a fit stomach was more than just a pretty six-pack. The exercises they created were designed to strengthen and protect the vital organs such as the kidneys, liver, spleen, intestines, and pancreas with a layer of muscle, in order to extend the length and quality of their lives and to make them leaders in strength, good looks, and longevity. Breath was always the foundation of this technique. We would do well to return to the ideal Bodhidharma taught his monks for human willpower and internal health and strength.

Since America's waistline keeps expanding, it is important to work on flattening the stomach. This involves not only ab work but also the strengthening of the spinal muscles to improve posture so that the internal organs are not compressed by slouching.

Start with one isometric ab exercise a day and then add one new exercise each day until you are doing five of them daily. Just by focusing your attention on this area for a minute or two a day, you will have better posture and a flatter stomach in a matter of days. The most important aspect is to breathe throughout the process. It is your breath that will carry nourishment to the abdominal muscles you are working and carry away all the waste products that tend to be stored in this area.

How to do it:

This exercise for flat abs can be done anywhere: sitting in your chair, standing, or lying down. Most people today must sit more than ever before (mostly in front of a computer), and this is one exercise you can do at work to transform your midsection.

Practice this move lying down to perfect the technique, then you'll be able to use it correctly sitting or standing as well.

• Lie on your back with your palms facing up or down, whichever is more comfortable for you. You may place a pillow under your knees to flatten your lower back. Because there are no joints involved in this contraction, you don't need the warmup. You can contract using 100 percent effort with each repetition.

• Relax your shoulders and jaw and inhale deeply. Breathe as deeply as you can, imagining that you're filling your entire body, right down to your feet. Exhale completely, and then take your inhalation into your lungs only, not into your stomach. Fill them, expanding your rib cage and chest. This is the classic hard-style breath, without the expansion of the belly, which is popular in yoga—a soft-style practice. Softly hold your stomach in and don't let it expand.

• As soon as your lungs are full, begin your exhalation and hiss while contracting your stomach muscles as hard as you can, pulling them toward your spine. This stimulates your internal organs. Exhale to remove all the stale air while holding your abs in isometric contraction. Make your stomach muscles quiver for about 6 seconds.

• Take three or more breaths while recovering. If you want to see a difference in just a few days, repeat this contraction two or more times. Relax into it and enjoy it. Next, try doing this exercise while sitting in a chair.

8. A BEAUTIFUL BACK

Every nerve that goes to every organ and to every part of your body connects to the spine. When you exercise your spine, you not only develop your back, but you develop your nerve force as well. Your nerve force is your vitality. The more you work your back, the greater your vitality. Your posture will also improve, and you can avoid the problems associated with a hunched back later in life. There's nothing sexy about a slumped posture. So, if you tend to look down when you walk, this movement will reprogram that learned posture, and you'll be one who looks up and straight at people, ready to take on life. This terrific isometric also lifts your chest.

How to do it:

• Squeeze the Orange. While standing, imagine you have a straight bar or broom handle in front of you. Grab the imaginary bar and pull it straight toward your chest while trying to touch your elbows together behind you. Tense hard and squeeze your shoulder blades together while you exhale and hiss, as if you were literally squeezing an orange between your shoulder blades. This one simple isometric exercise strengthens your entire upper back. It will keep your shoulders from curving forward and prevent you from slouching. Your back will become straight and your chest lifted, improving your posture.

• Superman. Lie on the floor on your stomach. Inhale deeply and stretch your arms out in front of you, like Superman in flight. Now exhale and lift both arms and legs off the floor, arching your back. Hold this position as you count to 6 and hiss. Relax and rest. This exercise can be a little challenging at first, but if you stay with it, it brings excellent toning to the whole spine. It is also a wonderful tonic to your kidneys. And it actually strengthens the pelvic floor.

You'll soon want to wear a backless dress, and you'll look far better in a bikini. You'll be happy with the fact that you have less back pain, better posture, and more visibly shaped back muscles.

9. THIGH SCULPTING

This is a great 12-second routine you can do while sitting at your desk. It not only sculpts your legs, but it also strengthens your lower back.

How to do it:

• Sit straight against the back of a chair with your feet 5 inches apart and flat on the floor. Place your hands firmly against the outsides of your thighs; inhale and press out with your thighs while you resist with your hands. Start with 50 percent effort for your warmup. Relax, then inhale again, pressing with a greater contraction, and slowly release as you exhale for 6 seconds.

• Now place your hands in between your thighs, palms a few inches apart and the backs of your hands against the insides of your thighs. In your warmup, try to close your thighs against your hands, using 50 percent resistance. Release, and inhale again. This time, use more of your strength to resist the squeeze of your thighs. Be careful not to press so hard with your legs that you overwhelm the strength in your arms. Work up to this maximum contraction slowly, since your legs are stronger than your arms.

10. SEXY, SHAPELY BUNS

This is such a good one that we saved it for last. Buns, glutes, bum, whatever you call them—these are among the largest and most powerful muscles in the body. There is no bone structure there to hold up the tissues; therefore, the shape of this area is determined primarily by the tone of the muscle.

Have you ever looked in the mirror and asked yourself why your buns seem flat and droopy? Why they seem to want to drop down to your knees even though you've walked for miles or done a lot of yoga? Have you wished for tight, sexy buns, especially when you're wearing shorts, jeans, or a bikini? Men notice tight buns; women often notice men's glutes at first glance.

How to do it:

• Elevator Lifts. Next time you are in an elevator (or waiting in line at the supermarket), inhale and contract your glutes *hard*. When you contract these muscles, you actually lengthen the lower back, which frees the nerves of your sacrum, one of the areas that supply energy to your sexual organs. Inhale deeply; tighten your buns as much as you can—*squeeze*—and exhale *only* at the point that you have begun to shake with tension. Release at the end of the exhalation. This is a strong muscle, and it can take the work and will reward you if you are willing to do this one simple isometric as often as you think about it. This will correct and enhance your posture and help to erase lower-back pain. This one exercise alone can save you a lifetime of lower backaches and a fortune in chiropractic visits. Squeeze and squeeze some more! This is the secret to tight buns, a happy lower back, and a much-improved sex life.

CHAPTER **7**

The Nutrient Advantage
USE MICRONUTRIENTS TO END NDD.

Every generation has the opportunity to leap forward with new ideas. It was a great leap forward in the 1980s when we launched the Information Age with the personal computer and the establishment of the Internet. We're leaping forward again today, with the ability to use micronutrients to end many of the symptoms of premature aging that lead to degenerative diseases. Micronutrients are the vitamins, minerals, and antioxidants that *should* be present in your food but are not.

According to the *Journal of the American College of Nutrition,* the amounts of nutrients in our fruits and vegetables have plunged dramatically since 1950. "Minerals like iron and magnesium have dropped more than 80 percent from our produce," says Al Sears, MD, a physician and natural wellness researcher in Royal Palm Beach, Florida. On his Web site, he continues, "If the soil doesn't have minerals, there's no way for vegetables to absorb them. And that's bad news for your health. Magnesium regulates over 300 body functions every day and is critical to heart health and healthy glucose metabolism. . . . In less than 50 years, the mineral, vitamin, and antioxidant value native to fruits and vegetables has been virtually 'destroyed'—robbing you of the natural vital nutrients you need every day."

A NUTRIENT RENAISSANCE

There is a renaissance going on in the field of nutrition and health, and you deserve to tap into it. Never before in history have we had the ability to identify micronutrients, isolate or duplicate them in the laboratory, and then manufacture them and test their effectiveness and safety. Even more important, never before have we been able to access the research that reveals their effectiveness.

Most of the vitamins that bring about the greatest reversals of the symptoms of premature aging were isolated back in the early 1900s. They were manufactured in the 1950s and have been researched solidly for effectiveness, safety, and required dosages for health and prevention from the 1950s to the present. This knowledge has not been made available to you, so you've been unable to take advantage of it. Just as a computer is worthless if you don't know how to use it, the censorship of this information prevents you from fully understanding the benefits you can receive from certain antioxidant vitamins and minerals. You had to be trained to use a computer. It is far easier to master the few key supplements that end Nutrient Deficiency Disorder and inaugurate a revolution in health.

Now you stand at a crossroads to break free and rise above the tsunami of degenerative diseases. The medical authorities cannot tell you that nearly every one of these diseases is caused by nutrient deficiencies. Their attention is on pharmaceuticals; they are racing to find drug "cures," and the costs to you are prohibitive when they do find them. In our population, nutrients in supplement form are taken randomly in most cases, but it only makes sense that with something so critical to your health, you need to know what to take, how much to take, and why. When you understand the magnitude of the benefits of the most basic nutrients, you can put an end to all the guesswork around supplements.

THE GREAT REVELATION

If you can pinpoint the problem, you can usually find a solution. Most of our experts are still running around touting low-fat and low-cholesterol diets; they are actually stuck in the dark. Those who seek answers in the thousands of costly new drugs brought to market, with clearly dangerous and very real side effects, are in the dark, too.

The pioneering leaders in science for the past 60 years have sought out good health in nutrients. These are molecular biologists, biochemists, and microbiologists who have watched the effects of nutrients on the health of our cells. As they heed the most commonsense and timeless guiding principle, "First, do no harm," they find that health is restored when the right nutrients are put into the body in the optimal amounts. Conversely, they see health in decline when people lack sufficient amounts of the right nutrients. These nutrients can be found both in supplement form and in actual essential foods. We will cover both of these categories.

You can either build youth or age prematurely—it's your choice. Your goal should be to end Nutrient Deficiency Disorder so that you can be anabolic, with the side benefit of ending this era of the diseases caused by nutrient deficiencies.

THE CORRECT PATH
OF PREVENTION

The nutrient advantage is our system for improving your health by using the *right nutrients* in the *optimal amounts* for *optimal health*. It's no longer acceptable to settle for less than the best! Thousands of studies that show the advantages of nutrients would make for very good news stories, but you don't get to read them because they're censored. While we reveal those that can help you the most now, you can expect grumblings and attacks from the pharmaceutical industry. The bottom line is, doctors and the pharmaceutical industry don't profit if you are staying well through nutrition.

In the words of Bruce Ames, PhD, of the University of California, Berkeley, in a DoctorYourself.com interview, "There's nothing wrong with doctors; it's just that they have no training in nutrition and they're not very interested in prevention. So you get a disease and they try to give you a pill."

The drugs in that pill, as you know, carry with them many adverse side effects. By using the optimal amounts of the right nutrients for optimal health, however, you experience "side *benefits*." There are *no* negative side effects because you are turning for healing to the very molecules that make up your body. The side benefits from the essential nutrients are numerous, as are the dangerous side effects from drugs, but they're conditions you *want,* not ones you fear.

Here are just some of the common side effects from several popular drugs: clumsiness, cough, dizziness, dry mouth, diarrhea, headache, loss of appetite, blurred vision, loss of sexual function, hallucinations, upset stomach, dark urine, irregular heartbeat, short-term memory loss, painful menstrual periods, agitation, irritability, slow or shallow breathing, open sores on the skin, rashes, yellowing of the skin and eyes, muscle aches or weakness, seizures, runny nose, nausea, nervousness, hostility, constipation, lightheadedness, shortness of breath, depression, mood changes, hives, itching, signs of infection such as fever, chills or sore throat, difficulty maintaining balance, erratic behavior, disruptive outbursts, severe drowsiness, tightness in the chest, slurred speech, suicidal thoughts, swelling of the hands, legs, face, mouth, lips, or tongue, and coma.

That's frightening! In contrast, examples of side benefits from essential nutrients would include but are not limited to: detoxification of toxic food debris and chemicals, removal of heavy metals from your body, protection from radiation from microwaves and medical/dental procedures, happiness, greater optimism, youthful skin, tighter pores, a glowing radiance, fewer wrinkles and fine lines, stronger nails and thicker hair, a calmer disposition, less or no depression, better memory, sharper thinking, reversal of brain shrinkage, repair of the nervous system, healthy blood pressure, cleansing of the arteries, detoxification of the colon, normal heart rate, stronger libido, greater lubrication, harder erections, healthy thyroid, greater hormonal health, greater fat burning, less fat storage, lowered risk of cancer, shrinkage of lumpy breast tissue, and better prostate health.

You're in the driver's seat. Do you want to suffer from the side effects, or do you prefer to enjoy the side benefits? Progress is often stalled when it comes up against an entrenched status quo. The airplane was ridiculed when Wilbur and Orville Wright first invented it. The controlling powers of that era refused to accept that such a breakthrough could be real. They thought the invention flew in the face of every principle of science.

We're discussing the same kind of breakthrough, and the controlling powers today find it equally baffling. They may be clinging to an outdated methodology, but this is an idea whose time has come, just as it did for the Wright brothers, who flew off and enjoyed the rarefied air despite the objections of the authorities. You have the advantage of a new paradigm—one of stellar health through a shift in your focus to nutrients—to vastly improve how you look and feel. Experts may question how it can be possible that a simple, well-known, and affordable handful of nutrients can do so much to remove the symptoms and causes of diseases. We want you to show them that it's possible.

The proper use of five key supplements is one breakthrough among many that we offer you. You may already know about these supplements, and you may even already be taking them. But in all likelihood, you've never had the opportunity to learn why and how they can bring about such remarkable improvements in the way you look and feel. Together, vitamin E, vitamin C, vitamin B, iodine, and vitamin D form the cornerstone of what we call the Nutrient Advantage. You deserve to experience anabolism, the rejuvenation and regeneration of mind and body that it provides. We'll examine each of these in the chapters that follow.

CHAPTER 8

The Sexy Antioxidant

VITAMIN E IS A VITAL NUTRIENT FOR HEART
HEALTH AND MORE.

Your doctor tells you to take an aspirin a day to thin your blood by inhibiting the aggregation of blood platelets. But perhaps you've heard of studies that link this advice to an increase in the risk of fatal pancreatic cancer in women. Well, vitamin E keeps your blood healthfully thin, without any adverse side effects. In fact, vitamin E delivers a multitude of health and sexual health benefits.

What causes the improvement in sex? When your blood is thick because platelets are aggregated, the blood can't enter the capillaries, which narrow as you age. The capillaries of the eyes, ears, and sex organs are very small and require platelets to enter single file, not in clumps. So thinning your blood ensures that all of your cells receive more oxygen, including the cells of these vital areas. Vitamin E supports hormone production and is used for erectile dysfunction. Even though aspirin thins the blood, it doesn't demonstrate these same sex-enhancing properties.

Women who take vitamin E for at least 3 months may notice stronger sexual desire, more engorgement, greater sensation, better lubrication, and more intense climaxes. One reason for this is that vitamin E helps women produce estriol and progesterone to balance estrogen. If your estrogen levels are too high, you won't feel like having sex. For this reason, vitamin E is especially helpful when the cause of female sexual dysfunction is an excess of estrogen. A condition of estrogen dominance can trigger PMS-like symptoms such as anxiety, bloating, headaches, muscle aches, and mood swings. Taking vitamin E daily for three menstrual cycles will help relieve these problems. With vitamin E supplementation, a woman's body has a chance to keep the progesterone it needs for hormonal balance.

Before Viagra, vitamin E was used in Europe as a treatment for erectile dysfunction—with good reason. Most men who take vitamin E for at least a week notice more sexual energy and stronger sensations. The reason for these benefits to both men and women is that vitamin E mediates nitric oxide production. This creates the more pleasurable sensations in women as well as in men.

In addition to enhancing sexual pleasure, vitamin E can boost fertility and potency. And here's more sexy news: You can also watch the quality of your skin improve. Your hair will thicken and improve in strength and quality, and your nails will strengthen to reflect your improvement in health.

THERE'S NO SEX IF YOUR HEART ISN'T HEALTHY

The best form of natural vitamin E is wheat germ oil, which has remarkable side benefits beyond improving your sex life. This is important to know. One out of four people in the United States will die from heart disease. Cases of diabetes are expected to double or triple in the next four decades. If you are diagnosed with diabetes, you have a 76 percent increase in your risk of heart attack, because the moment your blood sugar goes out of control during stress or because you have not eaten correctly or monitored your insulin, your blood may thicken so rapidly with sugar that your heart can stop. This, of course, is our firsthand experience.

Fortunately, wheat germ oil can help prevent such a catastrophe. We are thankful to have been able to unearth the following monumental research on how to prevent and reverse heart disease with wheat germ oil. This research has never been available in the National Library of Medicine, nor has it been made available on MEDLINE. It's been censored. We're introducing this lifesaving information to you here because we have seen it work in our own lives. The nutrient advantage from wheat germ oil is simply too great to measure.

Studies that you can easily find in the National Library of Medicine and on MEDLINE have attempted to *refute* the proven benefits of vitamin E for heart health. Sadly, the methodology of these studies has always been to overlook wheat germ oil, as if deliberately, perhaps to protect the vast profits of costly heart medications, unnecessary surgeries, six-figure bypasses, and all the other technology and trappings of the billion-dollar heart disease industry.

HOW TO PREVENT AND REVERSE THE NUMBER ONE KILLER

Doctors Evan and Wilfrid Shute of London, Ontario, were the first physicians to realize that an adequate vitamin E status is vital to the health of the heart. They were obstetricians who were successfully using wheat germ oil to enhance fertility in addition to reducing blood clots in the legs of pregnant women, which prevented strokes. They correctly discovered that wheat germ oil would also prevent the clogging of the arteries to the heart and that a certain amount per day of wheat germ oil—the only form of vitamin E available at the time—was beneficial in reversing heart disease and in treating angina. By 1954, the Shute brothers had treated over 10,000 heart disease patients with miraculous results. As they continued their studies over the decades, they successfully treated, prevented, or reversed serious heart disease in some 40,000 people using wheat germ oil in doses ranging from 450 to 1,600 international units (IU) per day, or just 1 to 2 tablespoons of wheat germ oil per day.

Unfortunately, during that time, the Shute brothers were personally ridiculed, and their findings were rejected by every established medical journal. Their peer-reviewed and duplicated research papers were deliberately ignored or suppressed by the pharmaceutical-medical establishment for four decades. According to International Health News, "A glimmer of hope occurred in 1959 when the Food and Drug Administration (FDA) formally recognized that vitamin E was indeed essential to human health." But the FDA went no further than that.

The medical research conducted by the Shute brothers on the treatment and reversal of atherosclerosis and coronary heart disease with wheat germ oil addresses a cure and treatment for our nation's deadliest disease. This is one of the key steps you can take toward ensuring the nutrient advantage, because it's your vitamin E deficiency, among other deficiencies, that is causing you to be at risk of heart disease. So let's start by ensuring you're on track to prevention with this powerful nutrient.

We believe that the Shutes' work should be considered on a par with Thomas Edison's in discovering the lightbulb. Their contribution is that significant, since it addresses the nation's number one killer, and the longevity and quality of life of hundreds of millions of people. Repression of their discovery has tragically and unnecessarily cost lives and dollars.

[A note from the publisher: Rodale Inc. always recommends consulting your physician before making significant exercise, dietary, or lifestyle changes, including taking nutritional supplements. People who are taking anticoagulants (blood thinners and aspirin) should take vitamin E supplements only under a physician's supervision, as high doses may interfere with the body's ability to clot blood. According to the National Institutes of Health (NIH), high doses of vitamin E supplements in excess of 1,500 IU daily in natural forms and 1,100 IU daily in synthetic forms may increase the risk of bleeding, including hemorrhagic stroke. Vitamin E supplements may also interact with certain medications. According to findings from the large SELECT trial study reported in the *Journal of the American Medical Association,* men taking 400 IU of vitamin E per day may increase their risk for prostate cancer.]

WHY WHEAT GERM OIL IS THE BEST FORM OF VITAMIN E

According to the National Institutes of Health, *vitamin E* is the collective name for a group of fat-soluble compounds with distinctive antioxidant activities.

Naturally occurring vitamin E has eight chemical forms (alpha-, beta-, gamma-, and delta-tocopherol; and alpha-, beta-, gamma-, and delta-tocotrienol). These perform different actions and functions in the body. Tocotrienols, for example, have been anecdotally linked to the prevention of hair loss and the promotion of hair growth.

Wheat germ oil is unique in that it is the only natural form of vitamin E that contains all eight of these compounds. Each of these eight individual compounds has proved to have antiaging, antioxidant, and health-promoting benefits. Tocotrienols, which were discovered only in 1964, offer many benefits. These include the treatment and prevention of strokes, pancreatic cancer, breast cancer, prostate cancer, skin cancer, and diabetes. Studies on the benefits of the tocotrienols are ongoing. According to Barrie Tan, PhD, a former professor of chemistry and food science at the University of Massachusetts and founder of a nutritional supplement company, in the past 6 years the Armed Forces Radiobiology Research Institute has performed extensive research on tocotrienols as a radiation countermeasure agent. It is good news that the armed forces scientists are looking into a *nutrient* that protects us from radiation. This is important for countless reasons: to protect those who are undergoing nuclear medical treatments, such as routine x-rays and CAT scans or cancer treatment; for those exposed to nuclear plant meltdowns; for those who use microwaves to cook their food; and for all of us who must pass through security scans on a daily or even an occasional basis. We need to know how we can combat this bombardment of radioactivity.

No form of vitamin E that is incomplete or lacking *any one* of these natural compounds can give you the magnitude of benefits of whole, natural vitamin E. The eight compounds work synergistically. You won't receive such extensive side benefits from any other form of vitamin E, including the foods that provide it, such as leafy green vegetables, grains, seeds, nuts, and fortified cereals. Although you should eat the whole food sources regularly—green vegetables, seeds, and nuts, in particular—the freshness of the food, how long it's been stored and under what conditions, whether or not it's organic, how it's prepared, and whether it's been processed will all make it difficult to assess exactly how much vitamin E you're receiving.

The nutrient advantage always requires the *right nutrients* in the *optimal amounts* for *optimal health*. With the exception of wheat germ oil, sadly, most vitamin E products are puny synthetic versions of just one of the eight compounds, specifically alpha-tocopherol. The *synthetic* alpha-tocopheryl is only 50 percent as available to our bodies as natural alpha-tocopherol. You want the very best source for all the reasons we've explained, and it's important to mention just one more side benefit: Vitamin E is good for your brain. You see, your brain is composed of fats called lipids. It needs a fat-soluble antioxidant to prevent decay caused by free radical oxidation. You want the best-known source for this important protection: natural wheat germ oil. Disregard the inferior forms that are available. Unfortunately, many medical doctors have not yet caught up with the correct information. By now you know why: censorship. Doctors and researchers lack access to the complete body of research that exists on vitamin E, which is why we are writing this for you.

A PIONEER DOCTOR SPEAKS OUT

The late Abram Hoffer, MD, PhD, director of psychiatric research for the Saskatchewan Department of Public Health and associate professor of medicine at the University of Saskatchewan, Saskatoon, led the campaign to end Nutrient Deficiency Disorder and disease through optimal supplementation of the right nutrients, and carried the torch after the death of Linus Pauling. He was the leader in reversing mental illness of all kinds with high doses of vitamin B and vitamin C. He spoke out tirelessly until his death at age 91 in 2009. He was so lively at that age that he was able to write nearly until his final year, publishing his last book during the year of his death.

In an editorial titled "The True Cost of Cynicism," published in the *Journal of Orthomolecular Medicine,* Dr. Hoffer commented on the importance of vitamin E. He and his colleagues found that men and women who took vitamin E daily for 2 years had a 37 to 40 percent decrease in the risk of having a heart attack. In terms of saving lives, this would mean that of the 616,000 people who die from heart attacks each year, about 50,000 of them could still be alive.

VINDICATION FOR HEART HEALTH THROUGH VITAMIN E

In April 2005, a study in the *American Journal of Clinical Nutrition* noted that vitamin E, like vitamin C, is safe for long-term use in a wide range of dosages. In this landmark study, scientists at nine universities in the United States, the United Kingdom, Germany, and Switzerland agreed that the previously reported side effects of even high doses of vitamin E (1,000 IU a day) *simply don't occur.* Even taking 1,600 IU a day has no detrimental side effect on healthy people who are not on blood thinners. This study finally confirmed the findings of Drs. Evan and Wilfred Shute, who began their research on vitamin E for heart health nearly 70 years ago.

The 2005 study debunked the idea that vitamin E was dangerous, and furthermore, debunked the notion that dosages above 400 IU were dangerous. Like the Hoffer studies mentioned above, it even more

Marilyn's Message...

Wheat germ oil is available from Viobin in liquid form. This is the form we use because we find it gives the most benefit, being closest to nature and devoid of the processing of encapsulation. A simple search online shows how many companies sell Viobin's product and no other. Clearly, it is the leader in wheat germ oil manufacturing and distribution. We buy the 16-ounce bottles, and we each take 1 to 2 tablespoons in the morning and the same amount before bed. I take less than Rock, who always takes the larger amount and also supplements with wheat germ oil at midday. He believes wheat germ oil gives him an athletic edge, and because he's had cardiomyopathy, he feels he benefits from the extra spoonful. Since the majority of heart attacks happen in the morning, a few hours after waking up, the nighttime dose is critical. For those who don't like the natural flavor, which I personally find pleasant, Viobin also makes wheat germ oil capsules.

If you're taking blood thinners, aspirin, or planning to have surgery, you *must* check with your physician to make sure wheat germ oil is right for you. It's good to know that after surgery, topical use assists in more rapid healing of scars.

deeply validated the Shutes' research, which had been suppressed for at least five decades.

It must be understood that the Shute brothers had no financial interest in the use of wheat germ oil. The researchers were not sponsored by the wheat industry. They made no money on this supplement that they used so successfully. We point out that, in the 1940s, when their work began, wheat germ oil was the *only* vitamin E supplement available.

The Shutes' work has been largely denied and discredited, not only by individual doctors and researchers but also by prestigious universities, the American Medical Association, the American Dietetic Association, the FDA, the National Institutes of Health, and the National Library of Medicine and its online research sources, PubMed and MEDLINE. We couldn't find any US agency or publication with a pharmaceutical bias, except for the *American Journal of Clinical Nutrition,* that had ever said anything positive about vitamin E. To juxtapose the suffering of those who could have benefited from the Shutes' research on vitamin E with the profits received by the medical-pharmaceutical industry that destroyed this research is mind-boggling. And don't think for a moment that these two new studies cleared up this devastation. Doctors around the country and agencies such as the National Institutes of Health are still discrediting the use of vitamin E today. As a result, heart patients are being forced to take dangerous statin drugs and undergo unnecessary, and sometimes deadly, surgeries.

CHAPTER 9

The Most Essential Nutrient for Youth

VITAMIN C SHOULD BE CLASSIFIED AS A MACRONUTRIENT.

Every time you consume vitamin C, somewhere in your body you stop aging. Somewhere you stimulate repair. Somewhere you bring about detoxification. Somewhere you eradicate infection and prevent free radical damage. Somewhere your skin will clear up. You may see fewer wrinkles on your face. According to an article in the August 2002 issue of *Biological Psychiatry,* you'll have more sex and less depression, and you'll ward off serious disease. And all this is just scratching the surface, because vitamin C is a miraculous healing nutrient.

What is vitamin C? In our opinion, it should not be classified as a vitamin at all but as a macronutrient because it acts like an enzyme in its ability to stimulate a multitude of beneficial biological processes and because it contains the appropriate mineral cofactors. Vitamin C can save your life. There are over 40 years of research on the facts, and it's no accident that these studies have been swept under the rug because the research was performed via naturopathic channels rather than scientific ones. Once we lift the rug, we have the answer to ending the diseases that threaten to shorten our lifetimes.

Vitamin C supplementation could erase all kinds of diseases. In significant doses, it could cure the major killers of the modern world, according to the book *Ascorbate: The Science of Vitamin C.*

Humans, primates, guinea pigs, and several other species are unable to produce their own vitamin C. Other species produce this nutrient in the liver or kidneys, but somewhere along the way in human and primate evolution, there was a mutation, and we lost the enzyme that allowed us to carry out this process. All other intermediate enzymes are still intact to produce vitamin C. We've lost only the final step, as have gorillas and other primates. These animals must *continuously* forage for fruit and remain in locations where they have access to raw plants that contain vitamin C. Anyone who has a guinea pig for a pet knows (or should know) that they must give it berries or vitamin C for it to survive. The common wisdom is that guinea pig pets die young, but the truth is more likely that many owners just lack the knowledge to give them vital vitamin C.

Your body cannot make vitamin C for you, so you are in the same predicament as the guinea pig. You must provide yourself with vitamin C to avoid many dire consequences. Vitamin C deficiency is linked to practically all the serious maladies you can name. This makes it an essential nutrient. This understanding comes to us from the work of Linus Pauling, PhD, and many of his colleagues, particularly Albert Szent-Györgyi, MD, PhD, a fellow Nobel laureate. It stuns us that because of profit-driven censorship, vitamin C has never been in the nutritional textbooks as an essential macronutrient. Rather than a micronutrient to be consumed in fairy-dust amounts—60 to 75 milligrams, according to the USDA's dietary reference intake (DRI)—this is a food nutrient, and it should be considered along with the other two essential macronutrients we'll cover: high biological proteins and saturated fats.

We can give you a tablespoon of water because you're thirsty, and then we can say, "Okay, now your tongue is wet. That's the entire amount you need to quench your thirst." The reality is that you need water throughout the day in far greater amounts than a mere tablespoon. And you need vitamin C in greater amounts than the DRI and pharmaceutical science lead you to believe.

In his studies to determine the amount of vitamin C humans need, Dr. Pauling measured the body weight of other species—from rats to cats to goats—and found out how much vitamin C was in their blood per kilogram of body weight. That ratio, without exception, always translated into a macronutrient amount—the equivalent of the protein that you would find in one egg. The optimal level added up to somewhere between 10 and 12, or more, grams of vitamin C a day. When under stress, mammals that naturally produce vitamin C double or even triple that number of grams. So it bears noting that your daily need for vitamin C could increase, depending on the stressors in your life, and your body would make excellent use of the largest percentage of this amount.

The super-antioxidant vitamin C is nontoxic. Being water soluble, it performs its duties and then washes out of your body when you urinate. As long as you maintain the appropriate levels in your body, vitamin C will keep working day and night in countless tasks of repair and rejuvenation. Just as you have to take water (H_2O) throughout the day as a chemical your body requires, vitamin C is a carbon-hydrogen-oxygen nutrient that is also a chemical nutrient you must regularly supply. As a donor, vitamin C gives what is needed to fix a problem and then is flushed out. This is why you must replenish often throughout the day. The moment your body is out of it, all repair and healing stop. So when you ignore your continuous need for vitamin C, you're actually saying to your body that you're willing to put up with all the symptoms of

Nutrient Deficiency Disorder rather than ensure yourself the nutrient advantage. You're saying to yourself:

- Go ahead and break that capillary so I can have more spider veins.
- That's okay, I don't mind that crease on my lip or my chin.
- Let the infection spread. It's all right. I'll get antibiotics.
- Gee, I hate being so constipated, but I've always been constipated.
- The tumors will spread. But what can I do?
- Oh, another asthma attack. I have to cancel my tennis match.
- The stress is making me sick. Won't somebody do something?
- Air pollution and radiation are facts of life. We're all going to die from some cause.
- What's wrong with me? I never feel happy.

Vitamin C is involved in literally hundreds of biochemical processes, and you need to supplement it because no amount of vitamin C–rich food is going to supply enough for all the processes it carries out for you.

In fact, vitamin C can save your life because there are few people walking around today who aren't suffering from the early symptoms of scurvy. From prehistoric time until the 20th century, scurvy was one of our greatest killers, as has been noted by scientists in the fossil records of hominids. They were not able to supplement their vitamin C intake. We still have these problems, including the warning sign of bleeding gums, but today we *do* have the ability to supplement. As you take vitamin C, the side benefits are that you will have smoother skin rather than wrinkles, feel happy rather than depressed, keep your arteries strong, create stronger cells, and feel younger than you could ever imagine. Vitamin C is your dream come true. This essential macronutrient is your body's all-purpose, 24-7 handyman. And again, we're just scratching the surface.

Vitamin C is one of the most-studied nontoxic nutrients on the planet. The higher amounts that are actually required show nothing but remarkable benefits. Vitamin C has low toxicity and is not believed to cause serious adverse effects at high intakes. The most common complaints are diarrhea, nausea, abdominal cramps, and other gastrointestinal disturbances due to the osmotic effect of unabsorbed vitamin C in the gastrointestinal tract, according to the National Institutes of Health.

But since both Dr. Pauling's and Dr. Szent-Györgyi's findings were essentially suppressed, doctors today know very little about the necessity and benefits of vitamin C. Irwin Stone, PhD, a researcher in biochemistry and the man who introduced Dr. Pauling to the vast benefits of vitamin C, brought us the understanding of the critical nature of vitamin C in its role in the production of collagen.

COLLAGEN IS YOUR BODY'S PRIMARY STRUCTURAL SUBSTANCE

One of the crucial biochemical functions of vitamin C in the body's chemistry is the synthesis, formation, and maintenance of a protein called collagen. Collagen is your body's key structural protein, and it can't be formed, maintained, or repaired without vitamin C. Collagen is the cement that supports and holds your tissues and organs together. In your bones, it provides toughness and flexibility and prevents brittleness. Without vitamin C, your body would just disintegrate. Collagen makes up about one-third of your body's total weight of protein, and it is the body's tissue system. It is the substance that strengthens the arteries and veins, supports the muscles, toughens the ligaments and bones, supplies the scar tissue for healing wounds, and keeps your skin youthful, soft, firm, supple, and wrinkle free.

When vitamin C is lacking, it is the disturbance in collagen formation that causes the fearful effects of scurvy—the brittle bones that fracture on the slightest impact, the weakened arteries that rupture and hemorrhage, the incapacitating muscle weakness, the joints that are too painful to move, the teeth that fall out, and the wounds and sores that never heal. One of the warning signs of a vitamin C deficiency—what Dr. Stone called subclinical scurvy—is the common symptom of bleeding gums. Because a vitamin C deficiency results in poor-quality collagen, suboptimal or minimal amounts of vitamin C over prolonged periods during childhood and early adulthood may be a factor that influences the high incidence of later-life problems such as arthritis and joint diseases, broken hips, heart and vascular diseases that cause sudden death, and the strokes that bring on senility.

Collagen is intimately connected with the entire aging process. Studies show that as you age, you need larger amounts of vitamin C to maintain and repair collagen damage from stressors in the environment such as pollution, ultraviolet light, CAT scans and other radiation, oxidative stress from free radical formation, and the harmful effects of the protein- and fat-deficient high-carbohydrate and high-sugar diet.

VITAMIN C, COLLAGEN, AND HEART DISEASE

In an article distributed by the Orthomolecular Medicine News Service, authors Andrew W. Saul, PhD, and Alan Spencer report that

> collagen is the most abundant protein in the body, and forms into fibres which are stronger than iron wires of comparable size. These fibres provide strength and stability to all body tissues, including the arteries. Vitamin C is absolutely essential for the production and repair of collagen, and is destroyed during the process, so a regular supply of vitamin C is necessary to maintain the strength of body tissues. . . . Linus Pauling believed that . . . we do not consume enough vitamin C to maintain the strength of the walls of our arteries. He suggested that of all the structural tissues in the body, the walls of the arteries around the heart are subject to the greatest continual stress. Every time the heart beats the arteries are flattened and stretched, and this has been likened to standing on a garden hose thousands of times a day. Many tiny cracks and lesions develop and the artery walls become inflamed.
>
> "Dr. Pauling believed that in the presence of adequate supplies of vitamin C this damage can be readily repaired and heart disease is avoided. However, in the absence of adequate levels of vitamin C, the body attempts to repair the arteries using alternative materials: cholesterol and other fatty substances, which attach to the artery wall.

Saul and Spencer go on to say, "If high blood cholesterol were the primary cause of heart disease, all bears and other hibernating animals would have become extinct long ago. They naturally have high cholesterol levels. One reason bears are still with us is simple: they produce large amounts of vitamin C in their bodies, which stabilises the artery walls."

THE MEDICAL IGNORANCE SURROUNDING VITAMIN C

Many studies have shown that hundreds of ailments can be treated and alleviated with vitamin C supplementation. Yet doctors are unaware, so you are deprived of the safest solution. Instead of employing simple, affordable vitamin C supplementation to address these ailments, doctors wrongly diagnose and choose to treat symptoms with much more profitable drugs and surgeries.

We have said before that the plague of subclinical scurvy was impossible to eradicate before the 20th century. Here's what we mean by "subclinical": Everyone understands that a tire works only when it is properly inflated. If the tire were totally flat, that would be called a "clinical flat tire." If the tire were only half filled, then you'd have a "subclinical flat tire." Sure, it may roll down the road, but not very efficiently.

Before the 20th century, doctors didn't understand the cause of scurvy and had no technology to remedy it. Scurvy has caused much misery in the human population. Because of the work of Drs. Irwin Stone, Linus Pauling, and Albert Szent-Györgyi, and the forward vision of Hoffmann-La Roche, the original patent holder for all the vitamin C in the world, by the mid-20th century we gained access to the benefits of vitamin C in the form of supplements. Now you can buy vitamin C supplements in the grocery store just as easily as you can buy meat. This affordable treatment of hundreds of ailments and dozens of life-threatening diseases is at your fingertips. You only need to know that you need it as an essential nutrient, and then you will begin to see that what we're telling you is true. Here's one way you can begin to prove this to yourself.

If your skin is rough or itchy, or full of little eruptions or fine lines and wrinkles, increase your vitamin C slowly to levels that approach 10 grams a day and watch how lovely your skin becomes. You are using a powerful free radical scavenger and a collagen-repair nutrient at the same time. If the collagen in your skin has been damaged by free radicals or all the sugar in your diet that competes with vitamin C absorption into your cells, increasing your vitamin C levels to this amount or greater will result in not only smoother but also younger-looking skin with far greater elasticity! This is just one small example of the benefits of having enough vitamin C for adequate collagen production.

We witnessed this very exciting ongoing rejuvenation of our skin over a relatively short period of time.

Unfortunately, to this day most doctors hold the position that all you need of this macronutrient, which lasts only 4 hours in the body (or until it is flushed away), is the DRI of 60 to 75 milligrams a day. In the dark medical environment surrounding vitamin C, you may also hear from doctors that vitamin C causes kidney stones. This is a myth! Totally false! Disproved!

There is a way to bring this macronutrient into your life to enhance all the hundreds of biochemical processes it performs for you. You must acclimate your body to its optimal dose. For you, this may be lower or higher than for others. Each of us has his or her own level. And this can vary depending on our size, stress, and environment, but there are some clear guidelines you can follow. If you smoke, or if you live in a polluted city and breathe fumes as you head for the subway and you follow the doctor's orders of 60 to 75 milligrams a day, that amount could be wiped out in your first breath of smoke or pollution. If you are a sugar addict, what you're doing to your vitamin C level is like making a deposit with the teller inside the bank, then going to the drive-through window and taking out a greater amount.

In supplementation, look for buffered vitamin C and take it with meals. Start slowly, increasing over 4 weeks to 3,000 to 5,000 milligrams per day. Increase your dosage slowly, after every meal, each week; take 250 to 500 milligrams the first week, then 1,000 milligrams the second week, and then 2,000 milligrams the third week. You will begin to have a greater feeling of well-being at this level as your body begins to detoxify and repair. Then keep increasing slowly to the 10,000-milligram level, if your body accepts this amount. You'll know your body's not accepting this amount if you start to feel worse instead of better. It will be different for each of us. Some can absorb far higher doses of vitamin C than others. As you take higher doses, let your instincts and personal research guide you further. As Dr. Pauling said, "Never put your trust in anything but your own intellect . . . always think for yourself."

Dr. Pauling was still actively lecturing at age 92. He had radiant skin and the most youthful voice and smile. He was not weak, nor was he in a wheelchair. He was taking 18,000 milligrams of vitamin C a day. He had cancer, so this dosage was relevant to him and backed up by his decades of research.

Many fruits and vegetables are sources of vitamin C. To receive from 3,000 to 7,000 milligrams of vitamin C per day—a broad range in which you will begin to feel remarkable results, depending on your individual biochemistry—you would have to eat up to 100 cups of broccoli or 100 kiwis or drink about 80 cups of orange juice. In the event you might try to do this, your sugar and fat storage would be off the charts, and you would have a major case of flatulence and the runs. Advice such as "Strive to eat nine servings of fruits and vegetables daily because you will get a healthy dose of vitamin C" comes from the American Dietetic Association. This highly respected organization also suggests "doing your best to work more fruits and vegetables into your diet before taking supplements." Understand that this misleading advice comes from the entrenched dogma of the US government's DRI, which recommends only 60 to 75 milligrams of vitamin C. This minuscule amount is typical of the thinking of our health care system, dominated by drug rather than nutrient therapies. This system—the substitution of one symptom for another—denies you the nutrient advantage. Just as you buy quality eggs for protein at minimal expense, you can buy quality vitamin C supplements in large amounts at minimal expense.

VITAMIN C AND CANCER

In 2007, it was determined by a National Institutes of Health–funded study on mice that vitamin C might inhibit tumor growth. Dr. Pauling was 30 years ahead of his time. He had been the first to conduct a clinical study on the effects of large doses of vitamin C on cancer patients who had exhausted conventional treatments. He demonstrated that vitamin C not only helped to prolong the lives of seriously ill cancer sufferers, but significantly improved the quality of their lives as well. The medical community and the highly profitable cancer treatment industry did not welcome Dr. Pauling's findings. There was an organized effort to discredit him by the Mayo Clinic, which attempted to "replicate" his trials.

Whereas Dr. Pauling gave the high levels for cancer supplementation in an intravenous form, the Mayo Clinic made do with supplements in oral form. This is a crucial divergence from Dr. Pauling's work, due to the impossibility of providing sufficient concentrations of the quality of vitamin C he was using. The Mayo Clinic erred in its methodology at extreme levels. Its research was comparable to an effort to win a race in a Model T against someone driving a Ferrari. Both are cars, and that's where the similarity ends. This showed how misled the researchers were in their effort to replicate the data. They didn't even notice what level, form, or quality of vitamin C to use.

Even though the Mayo Clinic study blundered in its methodology and drew antagonistic conclusions about Dr. Pauling's findings, no attempt was ever made to replicate his study correctly. This raises the issue: Are other highly profitable fund-raisers deliberately ignoring an inexpensive, noninvasive, and nontoxic new treatment for cancer solely on the grounds that it doesn't bring profits to our health care industry? If a new drug were introduced that promised even a modicum of vitamin C's benefits for cancer, the cost would certainly not be that of vitamin C, and it would be hailed as a breakthrough. Are we really looking for the cure to this debilitating and tragic disease, or is cancer just too big of a profit center for drug makers to study cheaper alternatives?

In his stature as a well-respected scientist, Dr. Pauling is too luminous an icon to ignore. Pauling was his own subject. It's significant that he lived to the age of 93, in an active, highly rewarded life of service to your health. He will probably go down in history for removing both heart disease and cancer from our population, as his methods are eventually proved successful, just as he fought in the 1950s and 1960s to ban unregulated nuclear testing. Will you wait 40 years for entrenched medicine to catch up to his stellar findings, which can help you reverse many symptoms of aging—and possibly save your life?

10

The Brain-Boosting B-Complex Vitamins

YOU MUST TAKE THESE NUTRIENTS
IN SUPPLEMENT FORM
BECAUSE YOUR FOOD DELIVERS
INADEQUATE AMOUNTS.

M ainstream medicine has failed to examine the biochemical basis and nutrient therapies for mental retardation, learning disabilities, and mental illnesses. The time for this is long overdue. In the September 2, 2011, *Morbidity and Mortality Weekly Report,* the Centers for Disease Control and Prevention warned that nearly half of American adults will experience at least one mental illness at some point in their lives, and more must be done to help them.

Are you depressed, always exhausted, suffering from insomnia? Do mood swings and irritability make you so edgy that you snap at your loved ones or coworkers? Do you suffer from ADHD or have signs of memory loss that cause you to fear that you're developing dementia?

These are your body's signals. Sometimes they whisper and sometimes they shout. Here's what your body may be telling you when it gives you these signals: "I have vitamin B nutrient deficiency disorder!"

The story of vitamin B is long overdue, begging to be told. Dr. Abram Hoffer's enormous body of work on B vitamins for mental health has never reached the public. At the age of 91, this biochemist, medical doctor, and psychiatrist published his final book, detailing the correlation between a vitamin B deficiency and schizophrenia and other serious mental diseases. It was more or less ignored. The volumes of work by Roger Williams, PhD, too, are virtually unknown at a time in history when they could not be more urgent or relevant. Dr. Williams retired from the University of Texas in 1986 at the age of 92. The active longevity of Drs. Hoffer and Williams should give you a clue about the mental and physical benefits of B vitamins. Will you be actively working in your profession in your nineties? These great scientists and doctors of orthomolecular medicine, who struggled to be heard about nutrient therapies, were both doing so.

Dr. Williams was the author of *The Biochemistry of B Vitamins.* He was the first to point out that all people suffering from diabetes and alcoholism are deficient in thiamin and vitamin B_1, an essential nutrient for the prevention of disease, especially diabetes.

B vitamins may help to manage the side effects of stress and diminish these effects in the body. Your body always uses what it can of a water-soluble nutrient, and if there is extra, it's eliminated through urination. And the B-complex vitamin is a water-soluble vitamin that washes out

(continued on page 72)

DR. ROCK REPORTS...

As a boy, I observed that the local veterinarian treated dogs and horses in a unique way. He would give them vitamin B shots and say, "This will fix them!"

Sure enough, a week to a month later, with gleaming coats and filled-out bodies, the animals were transformed. Their eyes were brighter, and with tails wagging (in the case of the dogs), they seemed restored to life. I always remember wondering, "If it's so good for animals, why aren't people taking it?"

My experience with the B-complex vitamins has been remarkable. After I was diagnosed with late-onset type 1 diabetes at age 55 in 2009, my research shifted in the direction of how to fight this disease. First, I found that before prescriptions for insulin, a few physicians treated diabetes by having their patients eliminate carbohydrates from the diet. This seemed obvious to me. If high blood sugar is the problem, why add sugar to my blood? So I immediately cut out grains and potatoes, all fruit and sugar, and ate only small amounts of vegetables on a high-protein and high-fat diet. Knowing that my body would make only the carbs I needed through a process called gluconeogenesis, I knew I would have the glycogen necessary for muscle fuel, as well as the glucose for my brain.

This was the prescription, and it worked for me: avoid carbs, and powerlift to build all my muscles and keep my heart strong and my blood sugar low, since muscle burns glycogen as fuel. So I began a demanding strength-training routine to repair and rebuild my heart after my diabetic heart attack in 2010.

From the time of diagnosis, when my HbA1c test (the measure of the average amount of sugar in your blood over a 3-month period) showed near-death levels of 11.9, until 6 months later, using my carb-free diet and strength training, I was able to drop that reading to 6.2, just two-tenths of a percentage point above normal blood sugar! Then I discovered the vast body of research that Roger Williams, PhD, of the University of Texas had left for posterity on the nutrient prerequisites for people with diabetes. It took months to understand all of it and realize how urgent it was that I apply it to my situation. I began eating and supplementing the very molecules our bodies are made of and require constantly for optimal health. During the next 6 months, I took generous doses of B vitamins to ensure that I was getting enough of the thiamin I was lacking.

Insulin had always made me tired. I would sleep right after breakfast, in the afternoon, and shortly after dinner. For the first time in my life, I was moody and felt unhappy. Then, within just a few days of taking vitamin B supplements, I started to feel much better. I had energy! I didn't need to nap. I felt like my old self again—upbeat and optimistic. Feeling great with my morning and midday doses of four tablets of the B-complex vitamins, I suddenly began to detect a shocking symptom that some people with diabetes experience: I was going into hypoglycemia—the dreaded low blood sugar that can lead to a coma in people with diabetes who fail to vigilantly monitor their insulin.

Hypoglycemia in diabetes means you have too much insulin in your blood. It can be a fatal issue if not managed immediately. The quick remedy is to eat raisins or hard candy. I realized that something besides my diet and my strength training was causing me to have more insulin than necessary. I went straight to the doctor for my HbA1c test, and the same doctor who put me on insulin found that I had dropped my HbA1c from 6.2 to a remarkably low 5.5—meaning that I was managing my diabetes to the point that it was a nonissue.

My doctor knew that I had been on a high dose of insulin from the time of the heart attack, taking 100 units a day. She instructed me to go down to 25 units and then perhaps to 10. This was exciting! Astonishing! I cut my insulin, feeling so excited that I was making my own and didn't need it that I began to get cocky and tapered off the insulin completely. That was a lesson I needed to learn. My blood sugar went up, so obviously I was making some insulin but not enough. I went right back on a dose of between 10 and 25 units.

Here's another lesson I learned in this experimentation on my own body: Over the next 9 months, there were times when I would slack off on the B vitamins I was taking and cut my dose in half. Why slack off? I'm human! I'm not perfect. But when I cut my Bs, my blood sugar went up. It took me a year to convince myself— through trial and error—that as long as I stay with the higher doses of the Bs, in the morning and at lunch, I need to inject far less insulin. I have proved this to myself. What an important benefit for people with diabetes to know about!

I also truly believe that the B-complex vitamins are preventing some of the dreaded effects that people with diabetes face. Since they heal and strengthen the nerves, I am protected against retinopathy. I had a place in my foot that was exhibiting early signs of neuropathy, but it is gone. Certainly the public could benefit from more supervised clinical trials involving all that I've just described, and not just restricted to those who have type 1 diabetes but for those with type 2 diabetes as well, the most common and more easily curable form.

of the body daily, so taking plenty regularly is not in any way overdosing. There are no records of death from a B-complex vitamin overdose, although there may be side effects such as gout, heart and liver problems, blurred vision, nausea, and vomiting, among others. Compare this with taking aspirin or acetaminophen. Compare it with the use of sleeping pills, which the *American Journal of Clinical Nutrition* has shown to cause a four-times-greater risk of death in those who take them.

For someone with diabetes, taking regular doses of B-complex vitamins is most critical, but there are so many other diseases, conditions, and symptoms that the B vitamins reverse and prevent. Regular B-complex vitamin supplementation is the key for everyone.

WHAT Bs CAN DO FOR YOU

When your car no longer has gas left in the tank, it stops. Similarly, if you don't give your body the raw materials it needs, it will grind to a halt.

If you give your body the nutrient advantage with the B-complex vitamins in the amounts it needs, you may be pleasantly surprised to find that your body will be able to face almost any situation. The result will be that you'll feel the remarkable benefits of returning health and energy. You'll notice that you're suddenly free from tension, thinking more clearly, and far more alert. You'll crave excellence more than you have before. You'll feel less nervous and stressed. In fact, B vitamins are so powerful for mood regulation that they can legitimately be called the "happy vitamins."

The question is not "Should I take the B-complex vitamins?" but "How much of the B-complex vitamins do I need?"

The first step is to check off the symptoms you are experiencing.

- [ ] mood changes
- [ ] irritability
- [ ] nervousness
- [ ] fatigue
- [ ] depression
- [ ] headaches
- [ ] dizziness
- [ ] trembling

☐ loss of appetite

☐ insomnia

☐ sugar cravings

How many did you check? If you are like most people living a modern lifestyle, chances are you checked at least two or three symptoms. (Are you feeling even more stressed because you checked *all* of them?)

The second step is to realize that the B-complex vitamins are so important that they are one of the *few* nutrients the federal government mandates to be added to food. They're added in tiny amounts, never in the meaningful quantities that are required for the nutrient advantage. Yet they are so incredibly necessary for the processes that keep you healthy.

For example, all B-complex vitamins help the body to convert food (carbohydrates) into fuel (glucose), which is "burned" to produce energy. Naturopaths realize that a B deficiency causes fatigue and the sour moods that accompany fatigue that we just take for granted. The Bs also help the body metabolize fats and protein. In other words, without them, you're not assimilating the two most essential nutrients from your food. The B-complex vitamins are necessary for healthy skin, hair, eyes, and liver function. They also help your nervous system work properly and prevent brain shrinkage and memory loss. What is important to know is that B-complex supplement formulas are created because the B vitamins must be taken together in a balanced form in order for your body to use them correctly.

Experts disagree on the exact numbers of the known B-complex vitamins. Some say there are 8, and others say there may be as many as 15. The 8 you will find in most B-complex formulas are B_1-thiamin, B_2-riboflavin, B_3-niacin, B_5-pantothenic acid, B_6-pyridoxine, B_7-biotin, B_9-folic acid, and B_{12}-cobalamin. Others that some experts include in this complex are B_4-adenine; choline; alpha-lipoic acid; methionine; B_{10}-para-aminobenzoic acid (PABA); B_{15}-pangamic acid; B_{16}-dimethylglycine; B_{17}-laetrile; and B_{20}-carnitine.

Let's look at what each of the 8 traditional B-complex vitamins does. We also list food sources, but we strongly advocate taking B-complex supplements to receive optimum doses.

B_1-thiamin: This vitamin helps to support adrenal function, helps calm and maintain a healthy nervous system, assists in preventing

Marilyn's Message...

I've lived much of my life under pressure, taking on far too many tasks, relentlessly challenging myself to excel beyond requirements. As a child, I pushed myself to achieve the highest grades in school and to assist my mom with chores at home. I would return from school with my own plan to surprise my mom by doing all the family ironing.

I kept on pushing myself right through college, often getting very little sleep. Beyond my workaholic tendencies, I also suffered from insomnia. My sleeping 4 to 6 hours a night started in college in the early 1960s, when I was going for magna cum laude and the National Honor Society's Phi Beta Kappa. This limited amount of sleep continued into young motherhood, which lasted from 1967 until 1978, and thus became a lifelong habit. Before our discovery of the B-complex vitamins, the condition had become more serious. I could not sleep because my mind was restless, mulling over how I would handle the many personal life challenges that were the catalyst for this book.

Everything changed for me when I began dosing with the Bs. I sleep far more deeply. I handle things in a more relaxed way. The inner, coiled tension to accomplish goals is no longer present. I still have the goals; I just no longer have the tension. Sleeping more deeply, I look younger. I can truly enjoy my day. I feel capable, excited, and completely optimistic, having let go of worry. This former workaholic is far more well-rounded now.

Having this improvement in my mental attitude, acuity, daily behavior, and abilities come to me in my late sixties is dramatic! I have a sense that I've been struggling on the inside with this deficiency practically all my life. The B-complex vitamins have balanced me. I am a far healthier and happier person. Like Rock, I'm living proof of the nutrient advantage of B-complex vitamins.

and reversing diabetes, and is necessary for key metabolic processes. Since we store very little thiamin in the body, we can become depleted in as little as 2 weeks. A thiamin deficiency can result in a condition known as beriberi, which literally means "I can't, I can't." Children in impoverished countries who are diagnosed with beriberi are not unwilling but rather unable to perform well in school because of symptoms such as mental confusion and speech difficulties. However, we often don't recognize a mild deficiency in thiamin in our own classrooms.

One study by Ruth Flinn Harrell, PhD, involving 74 children ages 9 to 19 years, demonstrated the power of vitamin B_1. Half the children were given a B_1 pill each day, and the other half received a placebo. After 6 weeks, a series of tests revealed that the group given the B_1 vitamin improved in learning ability tasks by an average of one-fourth compared with the other group. Dr. Harrell worked to promote her theory that supplements could help children with learning disabilities from as early as WWII to as recently as 1981.

According to *The Nutrition Desk Reference,* thiamin deficiency causes loss of nerve function, memory loss, reduced attention span, irritability, confusion, depression, and even paralysis.

Food sources for thiamin include romaine lettuce, asparagus, spinach, sunflower seeds, peas, ripe tomatoes, cooked eggplant, Brussels sprouts, and mustard greens.

B_2-riboflavin: In addition to producing energy for the body, riboflavin also works as an antioxidant to destroy free radicals. The free radical theory of aging put forth by Denham Harman, MD, PhD, in the 1950s is today considered by many scientists to be the definitive explanation for aging. This theory explains that free radicals are unbalanced renegade cells missing an electron. They move in nanoseconds, and they will attack every cell in your body in an effort to steal the missing electron and rebalance themselves. Bruce Ames, PhD, at the University of California, Berkeley, and a member of the National Academy of Sciences, says that every day, every cell of your body is subjected to 10,000 hits from free radicals. The weaker cells succumb and become free radicals themselves, or they die. Free radical attacks damage eye, brain, and heart cells, mitochondria, and DNA, and therefore they contribute to the aging process, as well as to the development of heart disease and cancer. For this reason, the arsenal of antioxidants we provide to our bodies—especially riboflavin—will give us the nutrient advantage that protects us from free radicals.

Riboflavin is needed to help the body change vitamin B_6 and folate into forms it can use. It is also important for growth and red blood cell production. According to the University of Maryland Medical Center, symptoms of riboflavin deficiency include fatigue, slowed growth, digestive problems, cracks and sores around the corners of the mouth, swollen magenta-colored tongue, eye fatigue, sore throat, and sensitivity to light. Riboflavin is important for normal vision. Some early evidence shows that riboflavin might help prevent cataracts—free radical damage to the lens of the eye that can lead to cloudy vision. Several studies suggest that people who suffer from migraines may reduce their frequency and length by taking riboflavin.

Food sources for riboflavin are mushrooms, calf's liver, venison, cooked soybeans, lean beef tenderloin, spinach, broccoli, and dairy products. Synthetic Bs are also added to most cereals.

B$_3$-niacin: Niacin is also known as nicotinic acid. One of its alleged properties is its ability to help you relax naturally and get to sleep more rapidly at night. Another suspected benefit of niacin is its ability to greatly reduce anxiety and depression.

Niacin dilates blood vessels and creates a sensation of warmth, which is often accompanied by a blushing of the skin. This "flush," or sensation of heat, indicates your saturation point for niacin. If you take 500 milligrams of niacin and don't feel the flush, you may need to double your dosage. According to *The Merck Manual,* e-published by drug-maker Merck and Co., the chance of severe flushing can be reduced by starting immediate-release niacin at a low dose (e.g., 50 milligrams 3 times a day) and increasing it very slowly. An intermediate dose is 1,000 milligrams per day. A high dose is 3,000 milligrams per day. The high dose may cause jaundice, abdominal discomfort, blurred vision, worsening of hyperglycemia, and precipitation of preexisting gout. People with a liver disorder probably should not take high doses of niacin.

Dr. Hoffer explained, "Niacin is a vitamin, not a drug. It is not habit-forming. Niacin does not require a prescription, because it is that safe. It is a nutrient that everyone needs each day. Different people in different circumstances require different amounts of niacin."

Symptoms of niacin deficiency include indigestion, fatigue, canker sores, vomiting, and depression. Severe deficiency can cause dementia, diarrhea, and a condition known as pellagra, which is characterized by cracked and scaly skin.

On DoctorYourself.com, Andrew W. Saul, PhD, suggests, "It is a good idea to take all the other B-complex vitamins in a separate supplement in addition to the niacin. The B vitamins, like professional baseball players, work best as a team. Still, the body seems to need proportionally more niacin than the other B vitamins. Even the US Recommended Daily Allowance (RDA) [now known as DRI] for niacin is much more than for any other B vitamin. Many physicians consider the current RDA [DRI] for niacin of only 20 mg [currently 14 mg for women and 16 mg for men] to be far too low for optimum health. While the government continues to discuss this, it is possible to decide for yourself based on the success of doctors that use niacin for their patients every day."

Niacin lowers blood pressure and cholesterol levels without the serious side effects of cholesterol-lowering or blood pressure medications.

Food sources for niacin include tuna, chicken breast, salmon, calf's liver, halibut, venison, turkey breast, and beef tenderloin.

B_5-pantothenic acid: Pantothenic acid is essential for humans and animals for growth, reproduction, and normal physiological functions. It is involved in about 100 different metabolic pathways, including energy and the metabolizing of carbohydrates, proteins, and fats.

Food sources for pantothenic acid include calf's liver, brewer's yeast, sunflower seeds, mushrooms, yogurt, yellow corn, avocado, legumes, broccoli, and winter squash.

B_6-pyridoxine: Pyridoxine is used in the processing and metabolism of proteins, fats, and carbohydrates. It assists in controlling your mood, as well as your behavior. Also, according to Tufts University researchers, "Across the study population, we noticed participants with inadequate vitamin B_6 status even though they reported consuming more than the Recommended Daily Allowance [DRI] of vitamin B_6, which is less than 2 milligrams per day." The author of the study also stated, "Three-quarters of the women who reported using oral contraceptives . . . were vitamin B_6 deficient." Smokers and the elderly are also especially likely to be at risk. Remarkably, even among people who take B_6 supplements, 1 in 10 is still B_6 deficient.

Vitamin B_6 is helpful in balancing hormones in women, particularly for women suffering from premenstrual fluid retention, severe period pains, emotional PMS symptoms, premenstrual acne, and nausea in early pregnancy. Mood swings, depression, and loss of sexual drive are sometimes noted when pyridoxine is in short supply and the person is undergoing hormone-replacement therapy or on birth control pills, although this hasn't been verified scientifically yet. Pyridoxine might also be of benefit to children with learning difficulties as well as to assist in the prevention of dandruff, eczema, and psoriasis.

A study of nearly 5,000 women by the National Cancer Institute in 2005 suggests that consuming more vitamin B_6 may protect against colon cancer. The researchers described the connection as "statistically significant." Any nutrient that has a "statistically significant" influence of reducing colon cancer risk is very important indeed. Almost 143,000 Americans are annually diagnosed with colorectal cancer and almost 53,000 die every single year (2008 data).

Food sources for pyridoxine include bell peppers, turnip greens, spinach, tuna, bananas, chicken breasts, turkey breasts, salmon, cod, halibut, snapper, and beef tenderloin.

B_7-biotin: Biotin is a vitamin found in small amounts in numerous foods. It assists in the metabolism of dietary carbohydrates, proteins, and fats, and it improves the body's use of insulin to help maintain normal blood glucose levels. In some studies, fasting glucose levels were reduced by more than 50 percent in rats given biotin!

Still under scientific investigation is the fact that biotin can also play a role in preventing the neuropathy often associated with diabetes, reducing both the numbness and tingling associated with poor glucose control. It is instrumental in maintaining healthy nails and hair, and it is used to treat mild depression.

Food sources we like for biotin include Swiss chard, tomatoes, carrots, almonds, eggs, onions, cabbage, cucumbers, and cauliflower.

B_9-folic acid: Folic acid, also referred to as folacin or folate, is needed for DNA synthesis and cell growth. It is important in forming red blood cells and producing energy, as well as in forming amino acids. Folic acid is essential for creating heme, the substance in hemoglobin that contains iron, which is crucial for oxygen transport. It is important for healthy cell division and replication, for protein metabolism, and in treating folic acid anemia.

Folic acid assists in digestion and the nervous system, and it helps improve mental and emotional health. This nutrient may also be effective in treating depression and anxiety.

Symptoms of folic acid shortage include diarrhea, heartburn, and constipation. You might also suffer from fatigue, acne, gingivitis, a sore tongue, and cracking at the corners of your mouth. Long-term deficiency may result in anemia and later in osteoporosis as well as cancer of the bowel and cervix.

You've likely heard of the importance of folic acid to the nervous system of the developing fetus. A deficiency of folic acid may increase the risk of a baby being born with spina bifida or other serious nervous system defects. Folic acid is widely prescribed for all pregnant women.

Food sources for folic acid include romaine lettuce, spinach, asparagus, turnip greens, mustard greens, calf's liver, lentils, beans, beets, and cauliflower.

B_{12}-cobalamin: Also known as cyanocobalamin, this B is unique in many ways. It is called the "red vitamin" because it is a red crystalline compound. It is the only vitamin that contains cobalt, a trace element essential to our health. Cobalamin is required in much smaller amounts than other B vitamins, although higher doses are often used therapeutically.

Looking for more energy? B_{12} is also known as the energy vitamin. It is often used by older people to help prevent mental deterioration and to speed up their thought processes.

Cobalamin is needed to manufacture and maintain red blood cells, and it aids in the production of DNA, RNA, and neurotransmitters. It helps support adrenal function and may calm and maintain a healthy immune system. It is necessary for key metabolic processes. According to Edgar Gonzales, DMD, some symptoms of deficiency currently under investigation include a sore tongue, bleeding gums, weakness, confusion, depression, fatigue, apathy, loss of appetite and weight loss, back pain, loss of balance, decreased reflexes, tingling of the fingers, and ringing in the ears.

Vegetarians are usually deficient in vitamin B_{12} because it is not manufactured in any plants. It is found only in animal products, so a deficiency is more likely for people on a strict vegan or raw vegan diet. Food sources for cobalamin include calf's liver, snapper, venison, salmon, beef tenderloin, scallops, shrimp, halibut, and yogurt.

Anyone consuming alcohol or taking laxatives or antacids regularly should consider supplementing with vitamin B_{12}. Older people are also likely to need supplementation; they may have difficulty extracting the vitamin from ingested food, as stomach acid decreases with age.

SOIL DEPLETION HAS REDUCED B-COMPLEX VITAMINS IN FOOD

Now that you've read about the numerous benefits of the B-complex vitamins, you're probably thinking that you want to start eating more foods containing them. We've given you plenty of options, and this sounds like a logical way to get your Bs. After all, many doctors still often say that the best way to maintain health is to eat a balanced diet, including lots of fruit and vegetables.

The truth is, you can no longer rely on food to get enough B vitamins. Modern commercial agribusiness strips the soil of nutrients at an alarming rate. Some of the foods we eat now, like apples, bananas, broccoli, and tomatoes, have a tiny fraction of the nutritional value of the foods our grandparents ate 50 years ago. According to the Global Healing Center, onions and potatoes have lost 100 percent of vitamin A in just 48 years! Most nutrients in our produce are down at least 30 to 60 percent in the past 2 decades, according to HolisticHelp.net.

Most people want less expensive food, and business wants to turn a profit, regardless of the cost to human health. Farms use chemical fertilizers, pesticides, and herbicides to kill insects and weeds. They genetically modify their crops, changing their DNA, because these crops are supposedly better able to resist harsh weather conditions and tolerate the caustic herbicides sprayed on them.

In essence, these businesses have re-created nature! And research shows their attempt is failing. There are harmful side effects to genetically modified foods, both for us and for our environment. We are now eating a brand-new mutant crop that is worse than what it was trying to improve on and a far cry from the healthy foods of a generation ago. So are the animals and farmed fish that we rely on for protein sources. Incentives for industry to continue genetic modification are all about control of the food supply, profits, and power. And this industry is growing by leaps and bounds.

As for the food, once it reaches the manufacturing stage, the nutrients that are left are further stripped during processing. To create foods of uniform color and texture, manufacturers actually change the food's structure, depleting nutrients in exchange for the convenience of a long shelf life. How many times have you seen orange juice with an expiration date of 3 months later? Yet if you leave an orange on your kitchen counter, it will grow mold after a few days. You can store oranges in the refrigerator drawer for up to a month or until mold grows. So how natural is your "freshly squeezed" orange juice?

Sliced white bread is another example. Grains used to be an excellent source of the B-complex vitamins, but most bread is now manufactured in large factories. One famous brand produces more than half a million loaves per day! This mass-produced bread is soft, gooey, laced with chemical additives, and practically devoid of nutrients. It lasts a long time. It's so laden with preservatives and artificial ingredients, even insects won't touch it.

What about fruits and vegetables? It's the same story. Many soy, corn, potato, and cotton farmers are planning to rely on genetically modified plants to increase their yield. Fruits and vegetables grown on farms and orchards whose soil doesn't have the minerals they need will be nutritionally empty.

What can we do? Let's first create a national campaign for government subsidies for organic farmers and the lifting of many costly government requirements that make it impossible for the small farm to achieve organic status. Let's put an end to subsidies for corn! Corn is one of the greatest causes of pellagra. It's unlikely we can change our modern farming methods quickly, but in the meantime, we can avoid the worst of the chemicals and replace the missing vitamins and minerals through nutritional supplements.

Let's place our focus not on the problems but on the solutions. You've been reading about all the benefits of the B vitamins—the "happy vitamins" that remove stress and anxiety, balance your many body systems, convert food into energy, minimize and even eliminate depression, promote healthy red blood cells . . . the list goes on. Few Americans, however, are taking the optimal doses of the B vitamins to receive the following (and many other) benefits:

• **Reduce the risk of colon cancer:** A National Cancer Institute study of 5,000 women revealed that consuming more vitamin B_6 reduces colon cancer risk. A statistically significant correlation between B_6 and colon cancer reduction is a significant finding. Studies also show that vitamin B_6, B_{12}, and folic acid help minimize chromosomal breakdown.

• **Fight multiple sclerosis:** Research at Harvard Medical School confirms that nicotinamide, the amide form of niacin (B_3), is a key to the successful treatment of multiple sclerosis and nerve diseases.

Dr. Bruce Ames proposes the "triage theory," which could have enormous implications for human health. The word *triage* is from the French word *trier*, which means to sort, separate, or select. Dr. Ames's theory states that nature favors short-term survival over long-term life, and our short-term survival is achieved by prioritizing how our scarce micronutrients are allocated.

For example, to keep us from falling over from lack of iron in the heart, iron is pulled from nonessential sources. If this theory is correct, when we are deficient in micronutrients, we would trigger the triage response and pull micronutrients from other body systems to increase survival today.

In another example, minerals such as calcium could be drawn from your bones in a catabolic emergency, when some part of your body's cellular structure is breaking, as in stressful situations, leading to osteoporosis down the road. This would explain why age-related diseases such as heart disease, cancer, and dementia could be unintended consequences of survival in the short-term at the expense of long-term health. These mechanisms developed during evolution to help us survive. But they do not guarantee a healthy old age. As the body breaks down and is repaired in early years, the graver consequences are felt down the line.

Age-related diseases, including weakened bones, hardening of the arteries, and cancers, have all been linked to inadequate intakes of vital micronutrients. You can trust the concept of the nutrient advantage to prevent age-related diseases. Nutritional supplementation is effective and safe. On the other hand, pharmaceutical drugs kill over 100,000 Americans every year (including overdoses).

Think about this: All the cells in your body are created from what you eat and drink, not from any drugs you take. Most people don't eat enough nuts, seeds, vegetables, and organ meats to supply all the B vitamins we need. When was the last time you went through a day without sugar, processed foods, alcohol, or caffeine? Each one depletes your supply of the B-complex vitamins, unless they've been altered and B vitamins have been put back in.

The average person eats way too much food that is deficient in nutrients. And the fruits and vegetables they do eat have suboptimal levels of vitamins and are highly deficient in minerals.

The most common mistake people make is to not take enough of the essential micronutrients in supplement form. A small deficiency in even one vitamin or mineral can cause many different illnesses.

HOW MUCH IS ENOUGH?

You can determine how much vitamin B to take by starting with a standard 50x DRI tablet or capsule per day, then adding one capsule per week over a period of a few weeks, until your symptoms are gone. Always take them with food, and never take them later than with a late lunch. Our dosage may vary, but most commonly we take two to four at breakfast and one or two at lunch. We counsel you to move into this range of amounts slowly. In every step you take that is new for your health, be gentle with your body. In this case, give it time to adapt to the concentrations of nutrients that are required for the reversal of symptoms and for healing.

Nearly every disease is caused by a nutrient deficiency. Your nutrient deficiencies of today are your diseases of tomorrow. It no longer makes sense to rely solely on the SAD (standard American diet) for nutrients. For the first time in history, scientists are seeing the effects on our bodies of the nutrients we take in from supplements and food. This is the revolution that brings you the nutrient advantage. The nutrients are here, but it's up to you to use them.

Boost your brain with the B vitamin solution.

You can prove to yourself that the Bs can actually bring you far better health and greater happiness.

CHAPTER **11**

The Danger of an Iodine Deficiency

WHY YOU NEED MORE OF ONE OF THE SAFEST
ESSENTIAL TRACE ELEMENTS

The alarm has been sounded: The world's population is dangerously deficient in iodine. In developed countries such as the United States, nearly 74 percent of "healthy" adults may no longer consume enough iodine. What's ironic is that the powers-that-be *created* this problem by running a fear campaign against iodine in the 1960s that caused us to avoid iodine by using less iodized salt on our food.

From the 1920s on, iodine has been a staple for healing in medical practices. According to Nobel laureate Albert Szent-Györgyi, MD, PhD, the brilliant, pioneering researcher of vitamin C, any physician who was in doubt about a patient's symptoms would automatically prescribe iodine because it was such a broad and powerful remedy. Back in the day, iodine was used to kill infectious bacteria and fungus, heal stomach disorders (some that could lead to stomach cancer), reduce joint pain, combat thinning hair and dry skin, and relieve symptoms of low energy and fatigue.

When so-called experts of the 1960s and 1970s attacked iodine, they pressured bread manufacturers to remove iodate, a type of iodine, from their flour. Until that time, it is estimated that at least 25 percent of American iodine intake came from the flour in bread because iodine was added in flour processing. As a result of these campaigns against iodine, even today food manufacturers use bromide in flour instead of iodine.

The remainder of our iodine intake came from a variety of foods, including milk and shellfish. This was possible 50 years ago because the soil was still rich in minerals prior to intensive farming practices. In the past 50 years, as American agribusiness has failed to replenish nutrients in our soil, iodine depletion has increased 50 percent. Bromide is an endocrine disruptor that inhibits thyroid hormone production and also, coincidentally, blocks the activity of iodine. Bromide is so toxic that the entire country of Australia will not use it as a food additive. In addition, because aluminum, lead, chlorine, and fluoride are in our drinking water, and many people still have mercury fillings, any iodine you may have in your body is used up removing these *highly* toxic chemicals, because iodine is known to increase the excretion of such toxins.

Iodine is one of the most important trace elements for human health. There is no anabolism without it, because the hormones for anabolism—growth hormone, IGF, and some say testosterone, too—require iodine. Without iodine, there is only catabolism—your body slowly breaking down.

Your body requires iodine for healthy cellular and metabolic functioning. According to David Brownstein, MD, an expert in iodine deficiency and the author of *Iodine: Why You Need It, Why You Can't Live Without It,* "Iodine is the most misunderstood nutrient. After 12 years of practicing medicine, I can say that it is impossible to achieve your optimal health if you do not have adequate iodine levels." Dr. Brownstein connects iodine deficiency to breast cancer and other diseases of the reproductive organs, such as ovarian, uterine, and prostate cysts and cancers. Physicians like Donald Miller, MD, a cardiac surgeon and professor of surgery at the University of Washington, find that women who suffer from fibroid cysts respond well to iodine. Iodine signals death to cancer cells.

Every cell in your body needs iodine to function properly. Your glands—ovaries, testes, pituitary, thyroid, and adrenal, especially—need iodine for the production of hormones. Without adequate iodine, the breast tissue may become cystic and fibrous, according to the University of Maryland Medical Center.

We live under stressful conditions in modern society. This stress unbalances our metabolism. The thyroid gland's primary function is to maintain a balanced metabolism, but it can't produce thyroid hormone without iodine. When your thyroid isn't working properly, it produces less thyroid hormone—a common condition known as underactive thyroid or hypothyroidism. You might have this condition and still not be tested for it because doctors can't see outward signs or symptoms of subclinical iodine deficiency. Meanwhile, you may be overweight, exhausted, and unable to concentrate. You may be suffering from cravings for comfort foods, such as carbohydrates and sweets. You may be cold when everyone else is hot. You may feel fibrous tissue in your breasts or have fibroids in your uterus. Perhaps your skin is dry or you're losing your hair. All of these symptoms are characteristic of people with iodine deficiencies.

Iodine may just be the most overlooked mineral, but its importance to health cannot be overstated. In addition to the need for iodine for the thyroid gland, when your thyroid suffers, so does the rest of your body. A major connection exists between low thyroid production and low adrenal production. Low adrenal, also called adrenal insufficiency, can actually cause someone's thyroid problem to be much worse than it would be otherwise. If your adrenals are low, your libido will go south because your sex hormones are low as well.

Marilyn's Message...

I accepted that my breasts would always be fibrous because they had felt that way as long as I could remember. After I supplemented with iodine, after just 2 weeks my breast tissue felt firm and smooth. This was the nutrient advantage at work: a profound experience of change for the better in my body. In addition, I began to look younger, to the point that I received feedback from friends that there was a significant youthful appearance to my face. Some people were speechless at the change. I attribute this to the effect of iodine on the production of growth hormone. When I looked at Rock, he, too, seemed suddenly more rejuvenated. It seems obvious to me, since growth hormone makes one look younger, that I was seeing this effect in action. There is very little debate today about the antiaging benefits of growth hormone, which your body can't produce without iodine!

If iodine plays such a crucial role in cellular health, why are we not being alerted to the studies that have been published? Why have so few studies been done? According to Dr. Brownstein, iodine deficiency is under-recognized because iodine cannot be patented, and therefore there is no incentive for the drug companies to perform the research. The consequences of iodine deficiency, Dr. Brownstein says, are severe: mental retardation, lowered IQ, attention deficit hyperactivity disorder (ADHD), infertility, thyroid problems, and cancer of the breast, prostate, ovaries, thyroid, and uterus. Adequate iodine levels are necessary for proper immune system function.

"More misery and death in the US may have resulted from [medicine's unwarranted fear of] iodine than from both World Wars combined," says Guy E. Abraham, MD, an expert on iodine.

To prove his point, in 1998 Dr. Abraham started the Iodine Project, a test on over 4,000 people to prove the safety of iodine supplementation. Here is what he found.

- Goiter is reduced or eliminated.
- Stress on the pituitary gland, which produces growth hormone, is eliminated.

- There is increased excretion of heavy metals by the kidneys.
- The liver's ability to detoxify the blood is enhanced.
- Obesity is more easily overcome; in fact, iodine deficiency may be a critical and unknown factor in obesity.
- Diabetes and high blood pressure are more easily controlled.
- Breast tissue normalizes, with decreased occurrences of fibrocystic breast disease.
- Menopausal symptoms are reduced.
- Polycystic ovary syndrome can be cured.
- Brain function feels less foggy.
- Heart function is better, with reduced arrhythmia problems.
- Cancer rates, especially of the thyroid and breast, are reduced.

Doctors participating in the Iodine Project found that patients who received sufficient iodine were often able to resolve issues related to diabetes without insulin. The doctors also noted that high blood pressure could be normalized without medication. This should have been front-page news! Millions of people suffer from high blood pressure and are on medications that create side effects, such as erectile dysfunction.

THE IODINE ADVANTAGE

There is compelling evidence that you can have better health, and avoid or reverse many serious health symptoms, if you simply consume more iodine. In the United States, a decrease in iodine intake, coupled with an increase in the consumption of bromide from bread, fluoride from water, and soy in the many varieties of so-called health foods that dominate our supermarket shelves, results in iodine deficiency. Soy foods and the soy feed in livestock block the uptake of iodine into the thyroid and have accelerated this epidemic of iodine deficiency. Let's compare ourselves with the Japanese to evaluate what we're doing wrong.

First of all, soy in Japan and all of Asia is not considered a prized health food or additive. It is simply a staple of their diet.

Second, soy in Asia is prepared in a lengthy and ancient fermentation process that we neglect to use in our country because of the added costs. Our highly processed soy loses the fermented components and inhibits healthy thyroid function, creates cysts and cancers, and interferes with hormone activity, as well as with proper cerebral and reproductive system formation in utero.

Third, how much iodine do the Japanese consume compared with Americans? The average American consumes 240 *micrograms* of iodine a day. In contrast, the Japanese consume more than 12 *milligrams* of iodine a day, which is 50 times greater. The Japanese eat foods that are rich in iodine, especially seaweed, including brown algae (kelp), red algae (nori), and green algae (chlorella). These sources are far superior to plants grown in soil, which contain only trace amounts of iodine. Saltwater fish and shellfish contain iodine as well, but you would have to eat 15 to 25 pounds of fish per day to get your daily 12 milligrams of iodine.

Let's make some important comparisons between Japanese health and our own. The incidence of breast cancer in the United States is among the highest in the world. In Japan, breast cancer rates have been among the lowest in the world—one-third of those found in American women. Life expectancy in the United States is 78.49 years, 50th out of 221 countries surveyed. In Japan, the life expectancy is 83.91 years. The infant mortality rate in Japan is one of the lowest in the world. They record 2.21 deaths under age 1 per 1,000 live births. We record 5.98 deaths under age 1 per 1,000 births—nearly three times as many. Coming full circle to breast cancer, in the United States today, 1 in 8 American women (over 12 percent) will develop breast cancer during their lifetime. Only 30 years ago, when our iodine consumption was twice as high (480 micrograms a day is one estimate), 1 in 20 American women were diagnosed with breast cancer. While there were other factors involved in these changes, it's obvious to us that iodine played a significant role.

Kelp is probably the most accessible, affordable, and effective form of iodine supplementation. One of its benefits is that it provides unique trace minerals that are found in the ocean but not in soil vegetation. Kelp absorbs all these minerals and locks them in, along with the plentiful iodine it provides. Typical kelp supplements are small tablets containing around 150 micrograms each. The dietary recommended intake (DRI) for an adult male is 150 to 1,100 micrograms. However, if you want to be more in line with the amounts consumed by the Japanese, you will want to take about nine tablets of kelp per day, three at each meal, although this would put you over the US DRI. You can also begin to take Hawaiian spirulina or chlorella, also rich in iodine, and eat far more seaweed in soups and salads.

A simple thyroid test will tell you if your thyroid is underactive (hypothyroidism) or overactive (hyperthyroidism). About 80 percent of our population suffering from thyroid disease has hypothyroidism, rather than hyperthyroidism. Once you see the test results, you can decide whether you want to go on thyroid medication for life, which your doctor may wish to prescribe. The problem with the common, less expensive thyroid medications prescribed by doctors, who wish to help you receive insurance coverage, is that they are the inactive form of thyroid supplementation T4, which must be converted to the active form T3, and many people cannot make this conversion.

We recommend that you discuss with your doctor a trial of a month or two of regular supplementation with the iodine-rich supplements we mention, with a follow-up thyroid test to determine whether you need more or less of these natural food sources. (Strangely enough, too high an intake of iodine may cause hypothyroidism, goiter, and other symptoms similar to iodine deficiency.) We believe that rather than worrying that you might take too much, the concern you must have now is that you may be taking too little. Although a study at the University of California, Davis, showed that overuse could cause arsenic poisoning, it's quite difficult to overeat on freshwater algae, sea vegetables, and kelp.

12

Solar Eclipse: Our Vitamin D Deficiency

TAP THE POWER OF THE SUN FOR ANTIAGING, YOUTHFUL ENERGY, AND PROTECTION FROM DISEASE.

itamin D is a fat-soluble vitamin that is difficult to get in sufficient quantities through diet. Because of this, exposure to the sun's UVA and UVB rays is the best way to obtain vitamin D. When the sun's UVB rays reach your skin, a reaction occurs that enables your skin cells to produce vitamin D.

Let's cut to the chase in this discussion. Adequate vitamin D is one of the great secret weapons against disease and aging. If you have high blood pressure or poor digestion, or if you have a challenge with your immune, mood, or hormonal function, you are aging too fast and you can be helped by vitamin D.

Why do we dream of vacationing on the beach among the palm trees and frolicking in the warm waves of some tropical paradise? Actually, this is a sexual dream, because exposure to the sun and its warmth stimulates two glands that play a role in sexual desire in your body: your pineal and hypothalamus glands.

The sun's stimulation arouses your desire for fun. You feel pleasure as the warmth of the sun heats your body and warms you from the inside out. You lie on a raft in the water or recline on a chaise longue and soak it up. The bronzing tan that comes from this sun exposure brings you a healthy glow, and you begin to *feel better.* You receive compliments on this healthier radiance. You feel less inhibited, which manifests first as a lighthearted happiness. Your focus turns toward pleasurable experiences. You feel better about yourself because your body systems are coming into balance.

When you feel better about yourself, you're more comfortable going out for a stroll in the fresh air and sunshine. You take pleasure in being out in public with your body less covered up. You're okay with shorts and tank tops. You're smiling, so people smile at you. Men flirt with you. Women notice you. This attention raises your self-confidence and your self-esteem. You are ready to participate more actively in life.

Obviously, we're meant to breathe fresh air and enjoy sunlight. The problem is going for an overdose of the latter. You need natural sun, with no sunscreen, for at least 10 to 20 minutes a day; and then you need to put on reasonable SPF sunscreen, such as SPF 30. We're not recommending that you go out at high noon for exposure. Early in the day or after 3:00 p.m. are probably better choices. Take a clue from gorgeous sun worshippers on the French Riviera. They break at noon for a long lunch in the shade of an outdoor cafe, take a siesta in a cabana, and then return to the sun in the late afternoon.

On the other hand, in this country, you don't hear this kind of advice. Instead you're told, "You have to be afraid of the sun. You have to cover up, slather yourself and your kids with sunscreens, and make sure you're out in the sun for only minutes a day. You have to make sure you're using the right SPF." Behind even an hour of pleasure in the sun lurks the specter of disaster: *You're setting yourself up for wrinkles, sun damage, and cancer.*

It's a dermatological message. You're told sun exposure is bad for you, but it's good for you! Doctors of dermatology and aestheticians keep the warnings against sun exposure front and center. It's never about pleasure in our culture when it's about the sun. It's always about premature aging, skin damage, and skin cancer. In our opinion, it's the beauty and health magazines that are bankrolled by the cosmetic sunscreen industry that are the first line of attack, advising you to fear the sun and to cover up.

THE REAL COVER-UP

What if you've been duped? For nearly 30 years, a collective group of individuals from dermatology associations, governmental regulatory agencies, and the media have been on a campaign to prevent healthy and safe sun exposure. What they want you to ignore is a historical fact. We've had a positive relationship with the sun for as long as humanity has been on the planet. Without the sun, there would be no life on Earth. For our entire history we've lived in harmony with the sun, not in fear of it. Only during the Dark Ages do we see depictions of life in a sunless universe. The paintings are mostly gray, painful depictions of suffering.

What you're not told is that scores of respectable researchers, epidemiologists, and dermatologists have published studies that show that sunlight is good for your health. It's as natural for you as food, and like food, it's necessary. Sure, overexposure to the point of burning your skin is not good for you, just as overeating is not healthy.

These researchers have predicted that if you follow the no-sun policy and the advice to cover up, the health risks due to sunlight deficiency could be far worse than any outcome from sunlight exposure. And the experts are right. Today we have a worldwide epidemic of diseases caused by vitamin D deficiency.

Let's put this into perspective. A study published in June 2008 in the *Archives of Internal Medicine* showed that men with low vitamin D levels have over twice as many heart attacks (2.42 times more). Now let's look at what this means in actual body counts.

About 133,958 Americans die from coronary artery disease–related heart attacks each year. And each year, tens of millions of dollars are spent to advertise that the cholesterol-lowering drug Lipitor reduces heart attacks by 39 to 60 percent. How many more lives could be saved by vitamin D, and without wasting all those advertising dollars?

Combined, all forms of heart disease kill over 724,600 Americans each year. These lethal forms of heart disease include cardiomyopathy, valvular insufficiency, congestive heart failure, arrhythmia, coronary thrombosis (a blood clot in a coronary artery), and coronary atherosclerosis (a narrowing or blockage of coronary arteries). According to the *Archives of Internal Medicine* study, there is *significant* reason to believe that vitamin D could help protect against most of these forms of cardiac-induced death, with the fortuitous side benefit of an increase in libido.

There are 1,255,000 heart attacks suffered in the United States every year. According to the American Heart Association, the annual cost of health care services, medications, and lost productivity related to these heart attacks is over $156 billion. If the only benefit of vitamin D were to reduce coronary heart attack rates by 142 percent, the net savings, if every American supplemented properly, would be (after deducting the cost of the vitamin D) around $84 billion each year. That's enough to put a major dent in the health care cost crisis that is forecast to bankrupt our country.

A reasonable question to ask is: Why doesn't our president, our Congress, the FDA, or the medical profession sound a national alarm for vitamin D supplementation?

THE WAR ON CANCER NOW HAS A WEAPON CALLED THE SUN

In 1941, the first scientific study was published showing that greater sunlight exposure resulted in lower cancer mortality. People living in northern latitudes were shown to contract more cancers than those in southern latitudes, where there is greater year-round sun exposure. Researchers subsequently identified vitamin D as the cancer-protective factor generated from sunlight. An article in the April 2006 *Journal of the National Cancer Institute* titled "Vitamin D Status and Cancer Incidence and Mortality: Something New Under the Sun" discusses cancer risk reductions of 17 percent and more based on higher vitamin D status. Numerous studies describe how greater vitamin D levels may reduce cancers of the breast, prostate, colon, esophagus, pancreas, ovary, rectum, bladder, kidney, lung, and uterus, as well as potentially non-Hodgkin's lymphoma and multiple myelomas. The evidence supporting the role of vitamin D in preventing common forms of cancer is eye-opening. Vitamin D–deficient women, for example, could have a 253 percent increased risk of colon cancer—*253 percent!* Colorectal cancer strikes nearly 143,000 Americans each year, and nearly 53,000 die from it. Another study found that postmenopausal women with the lowest levels of vitamin D were at a 223 percent increased risk for developing breast cancer. Most studies show that higher levels of vitamin D can reduce breast cancer incidence by 30 to 50 percent. According to the most recent government data, approximately 210,000 women are diagnosed with breast cancer in the United States, and 40,589 die from it. This needless suffering and death caused by insufficient intake of vitamin D is unconscionable.

Stroke is the number four cause of death in the United States. It is also one of the most feared diseases because of its high incidence of permanent disability. In a study published in September 2008 in the journal *Stroke,* German researchers measured blood indicators of vitamin D status in 3,315 people with suspected coronary artery disease. The subjects were followed for $7\frac{3}{4}$ years. For every small decrease in blood indicators of vitamin D status, there was a startling increase in the number of fatal strokes. A growing body of science suggests that vitamin D may have an effect on cardiac health. For example, a Harvard Medical School study published that same year in *Circulation,* the journal of the American Heart Association, found that people with low vitamin D levels had about a 60 percent higher risk of heart attack, heart failure, or stroke compared with people who had higher levels of D in their blood, even when well-known cardiovascular risk factors such as diabetes and high blood pressure were taken into account. If all vitamin D did was reduce stroke risk, it would be critical for every American to ensure optimal blood levels.

Vitamin D deficiency is a worldwide problem. Yet no medical organization or governmental body has declared a health emergency to warn the public about the urgency of achieving sufficient vitamin D blood levels.

Doctors today would recognize a vitamin D deficiency more easily if presented with a patient with rickets or osteomalacia (both diseases involving softening of the bones). Clinical vitamin D deficiency is diagnosed when blood levels of a vitamin D metabolite (25-hydroxy vitamin D) drop below 12 nanograms per milliliter (ng/ml). However, optimal blood levels of vitamin D *between 30 and 50 ng/ml or higher* are what some experts recommend. People with blood levels below 30 ng/ml are considered to have insufficient vitamin D. No wonder our doctors are at a loss to understand the widespread health problems created by less than optimal vitamin D levels. If physicians view a patient's medical chart and see a vitamin D blood level of 18 ng/ml, they might think this person has adequate vitamin D, because it's at the high end of "inadequate." A vitamin D blood level this low could make this patient susceptible to many of the diseases of aging and may in fact be the reason that individual has become a "patient" in the first place.

We believe that there is clearly a need for a new consensus in the medical community to redefine vitamin D deficiency in light of the new information.

THE IMPORTANCE OF VITAMIN D IN YOUR LIFE

Vitamin D is a vitamin you take in a pill or capsule. It is also the most powerful steroid hormone activated within your body from sunlight exposure. While you take your supplement, realize that the most natural and valuable form comes from sensible sun exposure. For us, a once-a-day sunbath of 40 minutes (20 minutes per side) between 9:00 and 11:00 a.m. works well, or after 2:00 p.m., unless we're in the tropics, in which case we wait until 4:00 p.m.

Vitamin D controls the genetic switches that guide your cellular life. These switches tell your cells when to grow, when to mature, when to divide, when to differentiate, and when to die. When your body has sufficient sunlight exposure, hence sufficient vitamin D, it has the amount it needs to trigger the appropriate genetic switches at the appropriate time. Vitamin D is an anabolic nutrient. It raises your testosterone and, some say, your human growth hormone levels as well. If you have a vitamin D deficiency, you may end up suffering from osteomalacia.

You are probably not aware that a Nobel Prize was awarded to Niels Finsen, MD, in 1903 for his successful use of sunlamps to treat skin conditions! And have you ever heard that dermatologists have used sunlamps since 1927 to successfully treat acne, psoriasis, and eczema?

Sunscreen is designed *only* to prevent sunburn. But we're an impressionable nation and believe the advertising that tells us it will also keep us from getting skin cancer. You can get skin cancer even without spending all day in the sun. There are other contributing factors to getting skin cancer besides sun exposure.

A DIFFERENT VIEWPOINT ON SKIN CANCER

Skin cancers can be serious, but for the most part, they are easily detectable and seldom fatal. In its later stages, melanoma is almost always fatal. However, in the early stages of detection, it can have a survival rate of 95 percent, or even as high as 99 percent, according to SkinCancer.org. You should know that there are some rather unusual statistics surrounding the cancer called melanoma.

- Outdoor workers have less risk of developing melanoma than indoor workers.
- Melanoma is just as common on areas of the body that are not exposed to the sun.
- Prior to 1955, melanoma was so rare it was not chartered as a separate disease.

These contradictory facts have caused a dispute between dermatology associations and some of the most well-respected dermatologists on the planet.

In an essay titled "The Skin Cancer Cover-Up," dermatologist Sam Shuster, PhD, states, "Every summer we're warned that the sun can kill. In fact, most sun-provoked lesions are benign, and not really cancers at all."

"There are so many misconceptions about the risk of skin cancer, that the entire field is replete with nonsense," states A. Bernard Ackerman, MD, author of *The Sun and the "Epidemic" of Melanoma: Myth on Myth!* He claims that there is no scientific confirmation that getting a blistering sunburn early in life sets the stage for melanoma. He also believes that the "more intense a person's sun exposure, the greater the risk of melanoma" remains unsupported, with epidemiological data on the subject proving to be "imprecise and inaccurate."

Sunlight is nature's way of providing us with our much needed vitamin D. And it's free!

An SPF 8 sunscreen will block the production of vitamin D in the skin by 95 percent. An SPF 15 will block production of vitamin D even more. Most sunscreens block nearly 100 percent of the sun's rays.

In other words, the common advice to apply sunscreen with an SPF of at least 15 a half hour before going outdoors is *absolutely wrong,* as is the advice to wear sunscreen all year long. By doing this, you're totally blocking the health benefits of sunlight.

The correct way is to experience 40 minutes or more of unprotected sun exposure during the morning or late-afternoon hours, when the sun's rays are not as intense. People with fair skin should start with 10 minutes and increase exposure gradually. Sunscreen should be used after this time to prevent overexposure and burning.

If you accept sunlight as your preferred method of naturally stimulating vitamin D production, then it is highly likely your skin will tan. The medical community will tell you:

- There is no such thing as a safe tan.
- A tan is a sign of damage.
- There are no benefits to a tan.

The fears are unfounded. Here's what you need to know that your dermatologist may not be telling you: The scientific definition of a tan is "protective pigmentation," or more simply, a protective sunscreen. In other words, a tan is nature's natural sunscreen. A March 2007 study from the Dana-Farber Cancer Institute states that the tanning process triggers genes in the skin to actively fight skin cancer.

Because vitamin D is free for the taking from the sun, and because it so clearly reduces all-cause mortality, many scientists and doctors, including Gregory Plotnikoff, MD, medical director of the Penny George Institute for Health and Healing in Minneapolis, stress its importance. "Vitamin D represents the single most cost-effective medical intervention in the United States," says Dr. Plotnikoff.

HOW MUCH VITAMIN D SHOULD THE AVERAGE PERSON TAKE?

If you're fair skinned, experts say going outside for 10 minutes in the midday sun—in shorts and a tank top with no sunscreen—will give you enough radiation to produce about 10,000 international units (IU) of the vitamin. Think about that: 10,000 IU of vitamin D in 10 minutes! According to Dr. Cannell of the Vitamin D Council, it is recommended that you take 1,000 IU per 25 pounds of body weight. A person who weighs 150 pounds would take 6,000 IU per day.

A fine source of vitamins D_3 is cod liver oil. Gel capsules can be purchased if you don't like the flavor of the oil. Vitamin D_3 is the specific form of vitamin D that is created by humans when the skin is exposed to UVB rays from sunlight.

Vitamin D is remarkably safe. In the *Journal of Orthomolecular Medicine,* Andrew W. Saul, PhD, wrote, "The one and only vitamin D-related death I could find confirmation of anywhere . . . was not directly due to the vitamin, but rather to side effects of medication." The best way to be sure you are getting the right amount of vitamin D is to have your doctor give you a blood test called the 25-hydroxy vitamin D test. If your vitamin D intake from all sources is maintaining your blood level at the high end of 30 to 50 ng/ml, you have a good vitamin D status. If it is more than 10 percent below this level, we believe that supplemental sources of vitamin D_3 should be increased.

Orthomolecular physicians maintain that people consuming only the government-recommended levels of 200 to 400 IU per day often have blood levels *considerably* below 50 ng/ml. This means that the government's recommendations are too low and should be raised immediately.

[**A note from the publisher:** Doses above 10,000 IU a day are known to cause kidney damage, and today's report sets 4,000 IU as an upper daily limit—but not the amount people should strive for.]

PART THREE

The Anabolic Foods

CHAPTER 13

Saturated Fat: What Are You So Afraid Of?

UNDERSTANDING THIS SO-CALLED DEMON'S ROLE IN YOUR GOOD HEALTH

What do you need to know about saturated fat? Let's talk about a nutrient that has been attacked so feverishly for more than 60 years that you've been terrified to include it in your diet. The repercussions of this poisoning of the public mind are catastrophic. Saturated fat is primarily found in whole protein sources. Whole protein/fat food is a cornerstone of both anabolism and the nutrient advantage.

If you're deprived of animal protein and saturated fat, you're egregiously deficient in these anabolic nutrients, so you're increasing your chances of catabolism. Without adequate protein and the fats it contains, your body is deprived of the fuel and building blocks it requires for muscle growth and tissue repair. Believe it or not, this is the reason you may not feel or look your best. Your body is tearing down your own protein-rich muscle and burning sugar while storing fat because a high-carbohydrate diet causes blood sugar to skyrocket, and your body must get rid of what it can and store the rest as fat. When this happens, your body is becoming catabolic. Saturated fat is an "essential" nutrient. It's called essential because your body can't make it. You must provide it to your body in your diet every 4 to 6 hours. This fat that you've been taught to fear like the bubonic plague is the most efficient fuel for your body.

More than likely, as you read the words *saturated fat,* you immediately think about heart disease or obesity. This is the outcome of 6 decades of political conditioning at work in your life. Powerful forces in industry, medicine, and politics have forced this programming on you. We're going to help you deprogram yourself. Here's why.

1. This programming is the root cause of Nutrient Deficiency Disorder.
2. It has contributed largely to the epidemic of degenerative diseases, needless loss of life, and untold suffering.
3. It's false and fabricated.
4. It has trapped you, and most likely your doctor as well, in a lifestyle that inevitably leads to the killer diseases that are always stalking you.

It's also important to highlight that this programming against saturated fat is the leading cause of Sedentary Death Syndrome (SeDS). This is because a high-carbohydrate diet creates the obesity and energy swings that keep people sitting on the couch instead of being active.

YOUR HEART PREFERS FAT FOR FUEL

Since fat is a *slow-burning* fuel with 9 calories per gram, compared with carbohydrates or protein at 4 calories per gram, your heart prefers fat as its fuel. The heart receives twice the amount of fuel per gram from fat as it does from carbohydrates. This makes fat a far more reliable energy source. Your body never wants to run out of heart fuel, which is why when you overeat on carbohydrates and don't eat enough saturated fat and protein, your body automatically converts any excess calories to triglycerides (fat) and stockpiles the fat.

When you overeat sugary foods, which is very easy to do, the sugar is turned into fat, which is energy for your heart. But the problem is, when this happens, the sugars spike insulin and turn off glucagon—your fat-burning hormone. And you store more fat.

On the other hand, when you consume saturated fat, it's not stored as fat unless, of course, you eat more calories of it than your body needs. It *turns on* glucagon and fat-burning enzymes, such as lipase. This is your body's natural design. You are a fat burner. The saturated fat you take into your body will be used, not stored, and it will slowly burn for about 4 to 6 hours, keeping your blood sugar in normal range. Nature placed fat for your benefit in the original natural foods: eggs, milk, butter, meat, and poultry. The proof of its importance is that saturated fat is a major component in human breast milk. Nature didn't put saturated fat into mother's milk by accident.

According to highly influential books such as *The 6-Week Cure for the Middle-Aged Middle* and *Protein Power,* both by Mary Dan Eades, MD, and Michael R. Eades, MD, some reasons for making saturated fat part of a healthy diet include:

1. Reducing Cardiovascular Risk

Currently there are no medications to lower lipoprotein(a), a substance related to the risk of heart disease. The only dietary means of lowering Lp(a) is eating saturated fat. Additionally, eating saturated (and other) fats also raises "good" cholesterol (HDL) levels. Finally, we now know that when women diet, those eating the greatest percentage of the total fat in their diets as saturated fat lose the most weight.

2. Strengthening Your Bones

People (particularly women) begin to lose bone mass in middle age. We all know that we need calcium for our bones. What many don't know is that saturated fat is required for calcium to be effectively incorporated into our bones. Some experts suggest that we may need as much as 50 percent of the fats in our diet to be saturated fats for this very reason. Commonly, 7 to 10 percent is suggested by mainstream institutions.

3. Protecting Your Liver

Your liver will clear itself of its own fat content more quickly when it has enough saturated fat coming in. And, this cleansing will help protect your liver from toxins like alcohol and medications, including those used for pain and arthritis, such as anti-inflammatories. This cleansing can even reverse damage to your liver. A healthy liver is an essential element of a healthy metabolism.

4. Thinking Better

The next time someone calls you a "fat head," you needn't take offense. Your brain is actually made up almost entirely of fat and cholesterol. It needs this fat to function properly and to keep you sharp enough to come up with a brilliant retort to the "fat head" comment on the spot.

THE REAL VITAMIN A IS AVAILABLE ONLY IN ANIMAL FATS

If you are wrestling with the idea that saturated fat is good for you, it may help for you to understand the necessity of fat-soluble vitamin A, which is found *only* in animal fats. This is preformed vitamin A, which is essential for:

- The prevention of birth defects and to ensure normal growth and development
  - The health of your immune system
  - Switching on genes to maintain normal skin health
  - Proper cell growth
  - The prevention of age-related macular degeneration
  - Antioxidant activity

Even though vegan proponents and enthusiasts of the plant-based diet will encourage you to seek your vitamin A in the beta-carotenes found in plant foods, this may be a dangerous and irresponsible recommendation.

VITAMIN D IS ALSO ONLY FAT-SOLUBLE

Now let's look at vitamin D from the perspective that it is a fat-soluble substance that acts like a hormone to keep your bones strong. The tireless, progressive doctors in the field of orthomolecular medicine are aware of this fact, and it is because of their relentless efforts for over 40 years that the public is *finally* awakening to the need for vitamin D. This vital nutrient is required for healthy bones and optimal growth and development, and possibly also for the prevention of multiple sclerosis, osteoporosis, depression, the common cold and influenza, and reproductive problems. Several thousand studies now link vitamin D deficiency to over 20 of the most common cancers, including breast, colon, lung, esophageal, and prostate cancer. Some alternative and orthomolecular medicine specialists use large amounts of vitamin D to treat these cancers.

In geographical areas that lack adequate sun during long periods in the winter, traditional diets always include substantial quantities of butter and other saturated fatty foods to prevent the natural vitamin D deficiencies from sun deprivation. Experts who attack saturated fat are contributing to the high level of cancer and the above list of diseases in northern climates. If you're cranking up the heat in your house, eat extra butter as natural vitamin D supplementation. Like the French, put a dab on your steak. Cook fish in butter and you'll receive a double serving of vitamin D, since both butter and fish are high in this fat-soluble vitamin.

THE "WONDER FAT": CONJUGATED LINOLEIC ACID

If such a thing as a "wonder fat" exists, it would have to be conjugated linoleic acid (CLA). Conjugated linoleic acid is an essential fatty acid that cannot be produced by the human body. Scientists didn't discover the structure or properties of CLA until the early 1980s. Literally hundreds of studies done since then have revealed an almost unbelievable array of beneficial biological properties, including:

• CLA could stimulate protein synthesis and muscle growth, and it prevents muscle wasting when combined with creatine and whey protein. It's both anabolic and anticatabolic.

• CLA inhibits the formation of body fat, and it reduces body fat in your tissues.

• CLA could inhibit or prevent several cancers, including breast and prostate cancer. It may inhibit the growth of tumor cells and reduce the size of existing tumors.

• CLA strengthens your immune system.

It is estimated that the average North American's intake of CLA is only approximately 25 percent of that required for a "healthy diet," according to the Ontario Ministry of Agriculture, Food and Rural Affairs. So here we have yet another example of Nutrient Deficiency Disorder.

The ministry also claims that dairy products are the richest natural sources of CLA. The highest concentrations are found in homogenized milk, butter, and mozzarella cheese. They are also found in beef and lamb, and are more abundant in grass-fed varieties of these meats. Low-fat dairy deprives you of your daily allotment of CLA, robbing you of fat-loss and muscle-building potential, as well as cancer prevention and the ability to lower your blood sugar or to raise your defenses against infection. As this country eats lean, the American wallet becomes leaner from health care costs, but the American body becomes much heavier. Research has established 3.5 grams, or 3,500 milligrams, per day of CLA as the dose likely to lead to health benefits—a level far above most current low-fat dietary intakes, which are a mere 15 to 174 milligrams per day. Adjust your plate to contain at least half of the CLA-rich anabolic proteins and fats.

BUTTER IS A HEALTH FOOD

Give any child a piece of toast and he or she will invariably say, *"Mo' buttah!"* Butter is a valuable food, and it needs to come back into the American diet. Many of us still dance around it today as if it will make us fat, along with eggs, dairy, and red meat. It's ludicrous that you're advised and conditioned to send your kid off to school with a stomach full of corn- or soy-enriched cereal—now that both corn and soy are genetically engineered ingredients—that is loaded with high-fructose corn syrup and often dyed to look like crayons. But the government agencies and most medical doctors still condemn the idea that you might want to give your children whole eggs cooked in butter. This malarkey has been going on for over 50 years!

It's all so upside down!

Butter has been a staple dating back to the prebiblical era. Records of recipes for making butter date as far back as 3,500 years ago. Hindus have used butter for this long, and their writings are replete with references to the gift of butter. In the Bible, it is recorded that Abraham offered butter to the angels because he considered it a sacred food.

Butter is imperative for anabolism because it's the ticket for nutrient absorption into your cells. Butter builds you up, makes your cells strong, and protects you against infection and fat storage. So embrace it! Organic butter is preferable to commercial butters, which are high in pesticides and herbicides that were stored in the fat of the animal and now appear in the butterfat. Eighty percent of antibiotics used in our country today are found in commercial agriculture. This is one of the forces behind the alarming rise of omnipotent "superbugs," the antibiotic-resistant bacteria that cause infections and the spread of infectious disease. But don't let all this bring you down. Just take your vitamin C, iodine, and vitamins E and D and you'll detoxify your body and protect your cells with stronger membranes.

Commercial salt, the kind used in salted butter, is also known as sodium chloride, a preservative. That makes unsalted butter more healthful. Go for fresh, unsalted butter and use it with gratitude, knowing it's an anabolic food. You can buy imported butters from France, Italy, Ireland, and Denmark. We believe that the variety of farming practices and animal feeds grown on diverse soils is good for you and is reflected in these products.

USING BUTTER IN PRACTICAL WAYS

When you roast, sauté, boil, or steam your vegetables, top them with a creamy dollop of delicious, unsalted butter. A *big* creamy dollop! For example, steam broccoli or broccolini, add butter and some very good-for-you Celtic Sea Salt, and serve it with your breakfast entrée of eggs. *Look!* It's morning, and you've already eaten a big serving of vegetables. Steam cauliflower until soft and mash it with plenty of butter, some cheese, and Celtic Sea Salt. Put some butter on all your vegetables and kids will like them better. And when you add some freshly ground black pepper, don't be surprised if they say, "Wow, this is *really* good! Can I have some more?" The butter on vegetables enhances the flavors. With enough butter and other seasonings, your family will become vegetable eaters!

FAT SATISFIES

As you overcome your conditioned fear of saturated fat and begin to eat enough of it, you will experience satiety after you eat. You'll find that you are no longer nibbling and bingeing. When you ignore saturated fat in your diet, you ignore the proven fact that it makes you feel full, not hungry. The hunger that plagues people who have a phobia of saturated fat is a real phenomenon and causes the tendency to overeat carbohydrates.

Let's examine the common behaviors caused by the deprivation of saturated fat. Say you order a chicken Caesar salad for lunch. The chicken breast is particularly anemic in saturated fat, which explains why it's such a popular choice in our fat-phobic era. So, 2 hours later you're hungry, and you stop in for a coffee at one of the popular chains that also conveniently serve sweets. You emerge with a paper bag and a coffee, and as you sit outside, chatting with a friend, you continually plunge your hand into the bag, pulling out bite-size portions of a gooey treat. If it's in the bag, you're not really eating all of it, right? Wrong!

Are you one of the people who won't touch bread, potatoes, or pasta, but while you're making dinner, your hand keeps finding its way into the snack drawer for pretzels, crackers, and popcorn because hunger is ravaging your system? You missed out on the satiety factor by eating that salad and chicken breast.

Are your kids always snacking on this stuff, too? The best way for you, and them, to feel full and nourished is to eat enough saturated fat. Look at the unhealthy behaviors that the demonization of healthy saturated fat has brought into your life—to say nothing of the results in the mirror.

CHAPTER 14

Protein: The First Food for Anabolism

FILL UP ON THIS MUSCLE-BUILDING
MACRONUTRIENT AND YOU'LL TRIM
YOUR BELLY FAST!

The word *protein* comes from the Greek *prōtos,* which means "first." In this era, it is fashionable in many segments of our society to look at protein as expendable—as a nonessential nutrient, or one that can come to you randomly as you graze on grains and plants. But protein is incredibly important. The quality and quantity of protein you consume will determine how anabolic, toned, fat free, and youthful you become. When you look at a person with a normal muscle-to-fat ratio, you see primarily a high-quality protein structure. When you see a person with more fat than muscle, or one who is in a state of bony emaciation, you see protein deficiency. Eating other foods at the expense of quality protein causes both.

Protein is a major component of every cell in your body. The amino acids in protein are the building blocks of any living organism. Proteins constitute life. It's highly important to our hemoglobin, neurotransmitters, hair, nails, bone, teeth, skin, ligaments, tendons, and muscles. If you're thinking about your appearance specifically, everything that people can see about your body is made from protein. Your shapeliness and tone, your eyes, skin, hair and nails, eyelashes, eyebrows, teeth—all of these represent visible protein. To look and feel your best, you must make sure you have plenty of protein, but not just any protein. If you want to remain young, you want to emphasize what are called the high biological value proteins in your diet.

HIGH BIOLOGICAL VALUE PROTEIN

Not all proteins are equal. Although protein is the most anabolic food, there are variations in the biological value to your body of the many different protein options. Biological value is based on three criteria.

1. How much of that particular protein can your body absorb to fulfill its needs of anabolism?

2. Does the protein in question contain sufficient amounts of the nine essential amino acids necessary for protein synthesis?

3. Does the protein contain saturated fat? If so, this makes it anabolic, which makes you youthful.

Protein synthesis is the process by which the liver converts the proteins you eat into the nutrients of anabolism, known as amino acids. These amino acids repair and build all of your body's protein structures, including your cells. However, molecular biologists will say that you also need saturated fat to build your cells. That's also a given, as discussed in Chapter 13. In short, protein synthesis generates muscle. If this is one of your goals, and you also want to live life at the top of your game, you will want to supply protein to your body at every meal, meaning every 3 to 4 hours during the day. Also, when you snack, it's a good idea to snack on protein. For example, a bowl of yogurt, a protein shake, an ounce or two of cheese, or a hard-boiled egg are all good protein snacks, and all can be accompanied by raw vegetables, if desired.

Protein is the fundamental structural material of every cell in your body and is made from amino acids, but not all proteins contain equal amounts of these vital building blocks of anabolism. There are nine essential amino acids—"essential" meaning that your body cannot make them on its own so they must be part of your diet. You must provide them regularly for anabolism and to keep your body toned. We believe that your body needs you to supply these essential amino acids at every meal. Once in a while, there will be exceptions, because we all break rules. But remember that *you alone* are responsible for providing your body with quality protein. No one can do it for you.

THE BRANCHED-CHAIN AMINO ACIDS

Three of the essential amino acids are called the branched-chain amino acids (BCAAs) because they are linked like the branches of a tree in an important peptide sequence to trigger anabolism. These are *valine, leucine,* and *isoleucine*—and these are the gold, the most highly anabolic amino acids. When your protein source is low or lacking in these three amino acids, it can be said that this source is of lower biological value. Leucine is the most anabolic of the three BCAAs, and in anabolic foods it occurs in a larger proportion than the other two; but you must have all three BCAAs for anabolism. This is because the branchlike structure is key to their effectiveness in your body. The remaining six essential amino acids are histidine, lysine, methionine, phenylalanine, threonine, and tryptophan.

Say you're sitting across from your friend at lunch. She's eating a salad with lots of grated vegetables, such as raw beets and carrots, and she's feeling virtuous. She's eating minuscule amounts of protein. You, on the other hand, are having a steak salad. You're the one with BCAAs, because they are not adequately present in plant foods.

All species have their foods. Elephants thrive on plant foods. Cats love fish. If you're not getting enough protein, it would be a good idea for you to supplement with BCAA tablets or capsules; however, you need all nine essential amino acids, so supplementing with only the three BCAAs won't totally fix your problem.

BCAA supplements should be taken regularly before you eat, and each manufacturer usually suggests a dose, dependent on that particular formula. Even if you're eating some animal protein, as in the case of people who eat mostly fish and some chicken, you would do well to supplement with BCAAs.

Four of the top natural protein sources that are highest in BCAAs are:

• Eggs
• Yogurt and hard cheese
• Red meat (such as beef, lamb, bison, venison, and pork)
• Poultry (such as chicken, turkey, and duck)

These are the most anabolic proteins to bring your body back to its youthful tone and reveal the muscle that's currently covered by a layer of fat. There is also a place in your diet for fatty fish, such as salmon, mackerel, and tuna; less fatty fish, such as haddock, flounder, halibut, trout, and cod; and shellfish, such as crab, oysters, and shrimp. We eat all of these, and you should also eat those you prefer. But we make sure that we eat most of the top four BCAA-rich proteins every day.

You have another option for BCAAs: processed protein powders. You can find them at health food stores and vitamin shops. There are so many varieties on the market that it takes some trial and error to determine what kind will work best for you. We prefer those with natural sweeteners that don't cause insulin levels to spike, such as Stevia and Zylitol. Our current favorite contains a fast-acting, undenatured whey protein isolate that is microfiltered, and it also includes extended-action micellar casein from grass-fed cows not treated with growth hormone or antibiotics.

A protein shake gives you the opportunity for a quick high-protein meal. But don't go overboard. Your body thrives on whole, natural foods, and too much of any processed food is not ideal. Protein powders are supplements, and they are, therefore, artifacts, so we keep them to a minimum.

A day's meals of high biological value protein might include one to two eggs for breakfast—poached, soft-boiled, or fried—with vegetables and/or ham, sausage, bacon, or cheese. It might include yogurt for a snack. You might have fish for lunch, and for dinner you would have poultry or red meat, such as roasted chicken legs, turkey thighs, lamb chops, sirloin steak, or filet mignon.

THIS IS A HIGH BIOLOGICAL VALUE PROTEIN DIET

The higher the biological value of your protein choices, the higher the anabolic effect and the greater the chances that you'll be out of the grasp of Nutrient Deficiency Disorder—and, as noted, the more youthful your body will become. The reason is that it's in these high biological value proteins that you find most of your essential micronutrients: the minerals and many newly identified and critical antioxidants. It's also in these specific proteins that you find the essential saturated fats that bring you the fat-soluble vitamins your body requires to assimilate protein. When high biological value proteins play the dominant role they must play in your diet, they turn on the hormone glucagon: your body's most powerful fat-burning hormone. Fat burning in this high-protein and saturated-fat whole-food diet is ongoing, which is what you want for anabolism.

In contrast, plant proteins that occur in nature are low in biological value because they are low in BCAAs. When you try to make them your only protein choice, the lack of BCAAs initiates catabolism. Unfortunately, for this reason, anabolic activity is difficult or impossible to support on a plant protein diet.

Marilyn's Message...

I learned about the importance of high biological value protein the hard way. I know firsthand about catabolism on the low-quality plant protein diet. I'm writing this book because of my traumatic experience after 2 decades on a plant protein diet. So when I share with you that plant proteins are simply subpar and inadequate in essential amino acids, I am speaking from my own direct experience.

If plants had adequate protein to create optimal health, I would not have suffered sarcopenia. My hair was thin. My nails would not grow, and they were peeling and brittle. The skin on my face was dry and lined. The skin on my body hung without tone, and my body sagged badly. Breaking down from catabolism, I was in a lot of pain. My knees ached when I went up or down stairs. They were so weak, I often had to descend one leg at a time. My neck, shoulders, and back killed me. And, even worse, my heartbeat was irregular, so I feared heart disease even though I ate practically no saturated fat and my cholesterol was very low.

Plant proteins are known as "incomplete proteins." As my vegetarian years went by, I was becoming an incomplete body, breaking down and in decline long before I realized it. Aging struck me hard in my mid-fifties, right after I wrote *Fitonics for Life* with Rock. This book was my first attempt to articulate a more reasonable maintenance program for Fit for Life, *because I needed one,* and because I was hearing from many of my readers that the vegetarian diet I espoused was too hard for them. I also had grandchildren coming, and instinctively I didn't want them to be raised vegetarian.

However, the transition I was explaining in *Fitonics* came nearly 20 years into an ingrained habit. I would go back and forth as Rock patiently made every attempt to convince me how much he and I needed protein.

As this condition progressed into my sixties, I became terrified of air travel, and I lost the confidence to drive long distances away from home. Rock would often have to take me home because of my anxiety attacks.

Something had to change!

I had to be educated about all of this before I was willing to change. I was committed to the dogma of the plant-based diet in the era before the Internet, when there was little access to the research that might prove it wrong. And the education took a long time to sink in because I didn't want to accept it. It was in such direct conflict with so many of my vegetarian beliefs. How could I go back to eating animals? I had to convince myself that this was what I needed through trial and error, going back and forth between a meat-based and a plant-based diet, until I discovered I was making progress in healing myself when I was no longer a vegetarian.

When you live in a catabolic body, you tend to accept the way you feel as normal. I failed to recognize how hard my life was, failed to acknowledge the depression I was always fighting. I'd been there so long, I just thought this was my life. I was feeling old, and also secretly wrestling with the transition and the backlash from the vegan community, since I was the first to be questioning their lifestyle. And the backlash came after *Fitonics,* which contained my first rationale for eating meat.

The vegans were arguing against me that the amino acid pool allows your body to always find the protein it needs. It does! This is the definition of catabolism. The body tears your muscle down to create its amino acid pool. If you're only eating plants, the high biological value proteins are in such low quantity that you have to supplement by allowing your body to "eat itself." Even if you take branched-chain amino acid supplements, you're still shortchanging yourself. You need to eat protein foods.

You can't know how beautiful it is to be in an anabolic body until you experience it fully. This is truly the ongoing feeling of lasting youth. It's impossible to be anabolic doing what most vegetarians and vegans are doing. I'm sorry about that, but I finally understood that the lifestyle I practiced for so many years could destroy the body. The good news is, I fixed it all with the message in this book.

PROTEIN IS THE NUMBER ONE ESSENTIAL MACRONUTRIENT

Your body does not store protein. Your body requires it from outside sources every single day, every 3 to 4 hours. If your protein needs are not adequately met by your dietary choices, you face a serious disadvantage. The secretion of the stress hormone cortisol is triggered when your brain cannot find its required protein sources. Cortisol signals the breaking down of your own protein structures—your muscles first—for the amino acids your body needs to keep your heart and other organs and cells in good repair. If you're extremely deficient in muscle, imagine that your heart and organs are breaking down, because without protein, this is inevitable.

Some say that Yogis and Buddhist monks historically consumed low-protein plant choices to suppress their libido. Unfortunately, today's yoga teachers often recommend plant proteins to their students, creating the same results of low libido in an unsuspecting population. Low biological value proteins also create other mental disturbances. The inability to focus and put in hours of concentration signals a protein inadequacy, which is why many people take fish oil supplements. If you allow this to endure for long, you won't be chanting Om but rather OMG ("Oh my God!").

Do not embrace the vegan or vegetarian path late in life. Be aware that the elderly need protein to keep strong.

THE LINK BETWEEN ANABOLIC FOODS AND HORMONES

Your anabolic protein and fat choices work very well with your hormones. First of all, cholesterol, usually found in higher levels in animal proteins, raises all the fat-burning and sex hormones levels by being synthesized into these hormones. Second, the natural balance of saturated fats in whole proteins turns on glucagon—your fat-burning hormone. Animal proteins turn on human growth hormone (HGH), which stimulates the production of insulin-like growth factor (IGF). If you have an extra $3,000 a month, you can get a treatment in a rejuvenation clinic that will release HGH and thus IGF for 7 seconds per shot. Or you can simply eat adequate amounts of the saturated fat in high biological value proteins, which means you'll be stimulating these important rejuvenation hormones. In this way, saturated fat is also the ticket to prettier skin with fewer wrinkles. The cholesterol it delivers is the basis of every cell in your body, including the cells of your skin.

The adrenal hormones—cortisol, aldosterone, and testosterone—are made from the cholesterol that comes into your body along with saturated fat. Men, take note before you order that salad! This is also important for women who want to enjoy their sexuality and want to build muscle tissue.

We're giving you back your whole eggs, red meat, dark-meat poultry, butter, and dairy products, and any other foods like these that you gave up but would still like to eat. For those in the over-40 set, that means you're free to enjoy what you grew up on.

The proteins we've eaten since the beginning of our journey on this planet are the high biological value proteins. Whole grains came to us only 10,000 years ago with the agrarian age, and processed grains and sugars didn't arrive in any abundance in the West until the 1920s. We ate mostly whole proteins in the form of eggs, dairy, meat, poultry, and fish until less than 100 years ago. There are plenty of studies that show that a low-protein diet causes substantially lower zinc and testosterone levels for men, leading to a far higher risk of erectile dysfunction and impotence.

THE MOST SERIOUS PROBLEMS WITH SOY

Since we've covered the whole natural fats and proteins that end Nutrient Deficiency Disorder, we may as well touch on one extremely popular protein option today that should not be consumed. This is soy. There is plenty of peer-reviewed research that shows that eating only soy may be linked to zinc deficiency, hypothyroidism, breast cancer, infertility, impotence, defects in the formation of the reproductive systems of unborn children, and dementia. When the FDA commissioner gave the soy industry her "heart healthy" blessing, she overruled the protests of FDA scientists who were afraid that the public would be misled into thinking that soy products were healthy in all respects, and not just for lowering cholesterol.

Many issues arise with this popular "health" food that Americans consume "virtuously" because it is considered sustainable and humane. One problem with soy is that we don't prepare it using the complicated fermenting process that's been the traditional method in Asia for thousands of years. This time-consuming method of correct preparation would dramatically lower profits for the soy industry in our country. The result is that our commercial soy is an unhealthy processed food. Soy milk is almost always adulterated with sugar and flavorings because it tastes so bad (to us, anyway). Soy meat and cheese analogues are adulterated with dozens of forms of MSG. Soy contains enzyme inhibitors that prevent adequate protein synthesis and phytates that prevent the absorption of zinc. When you eat meat with soy, the soy will block your ability to absorb the amino acids and zinc in the meat.

Most soy in the United States is genetically modified—up to 91 percent, according to an article from NaturalNews.com, quoting research from GMO Compass. In the United States, 60 to 70 percent of the food supply contains at least one genetically engineered ingredient. This is why people in the know read labels and put back any product that contains any form of soy. Genetically modified food should be labeled, but it isn't. The point we are making here is that soy is not a viable protein choice in the Young for Life program. It should certainly not be your first choice!

We aren't hearing about the effects of soy on vegans, who probably eat the most of this inferior protein source. What are they experiencing in terms of increased infertility, cancer, loss of libido, and zinc deficiency? Since the vegan diet took root in the mainstream as recently as the early 1990's, there are no long-term studies . . . yet.

CHAPTER 15

Surprise! Excessive Carbohydrates Cause NDD

THE EARLIEST HUMANS LIVED A LOW-CARB LIFESTYLE, SO WHY DON'T WE?

There is no such thing as an essential carbohydrate. There are essential amino acids, which make proteins essential. There are essential fatty acids, so fats are essential. There is essential ascorbic acid (vitamin C). The term *essential* in nutrition science means that your body cannot manufacture it; you must supply it through your diet. The reason you need to supply only low amounts of carbohydrates in your diet is because your body is designed to make just the amount of sugar it needs—no more and no less.

GRAIN WAS OUR FIRST PROCESSED FOOD

Anthropologists report that early humans lived on a low-carbohydrate diet. Their carbohydrate consumption, which was around 80 grams of carbohydrates a day, came primarily from the root and leafy green vegetables they foraged in warm weather. Today, health-seeking Americans who think they are doing something good for themselves, and those who are just bumping along on standard American fare, are eating between 350 to 600 grams of carbohydrates a day. If you're eating this amount of the sugar, it's bye-bye lean and sexy, hello fat and flabby.

Fat and protein have defined the human diet through the millennia. Our earliest ancestors hunted and gathered the small and large game, eggs, and fish that were everywhere around them. They used *all* of the game—fat, hide, and bones; nothing was wasted. The limited carbohydrate foods they did have—fruits or young, sprouted plants, herbs, roots, and tubers from the meadows—were available only during certain seasons. It was 23,000 years ago that the early humans began to process grain plants into cereal. These plants are not a food nature intended for humans. Too much has to be done to turn them into food. If you want to argue, as some diet commentators do, that we evolved when we began to eat grain, not so fast! We survived life in the wild without *any* of our modern conveniences. As we "evolved" into eating a carb-based diet, part of our so-called progress included the technology for cigarettes, Vioxx, and the nuclear bomb. Were we really moving forward? If you look at the facts, all these examples, including our excessive refined and whole grain consumption, kill, maim, and threaten our survival.

For most of our experience on this planet, we've faced starvation, not obesity, as a natural life challenge. Nature designed insulin as one of the first and most vital hormones for survival in times of starvation. Insulin is made from protein, not carbohydrates. This hormone delivers amino acids to your muscles, as well as glycogen for fueling them. But, when you overeat carbohydrates and sugars—whether they are whole or refined—and your blood glucose skyrockets, this is a totally unnatural emergency for your body, and it never could have happened before the elevation of grains as food.

In *The 6-Week Cure for the Middle-Aged Middle,* authors Mary Dan Eades, MD, and Michael R. Eades, MD, write, "Whole grains send insulin and glucose up a little less than similar dishes made with refined white flour, but it's still a big surge upward. And upward is bad. When insulin is up, you store calories as fat and can't access your fat stores for fuel. People with insulin resistance and metabolic syndrome, who have chronically high insulin levels, will sometimes pack incoming calories into storage to a degree that leaves them without enough available calories for burning to meet the body's energy needs. (This phenomenon has been termed malnutrition or starvation in the face of plenty—i.e., there is plenty of energy in the account; you just don't have the password to access it.)"

This explains obesity, and why high blood sugar was much less prevalent 100 years ago. It was nearly impossible to have high blood sugar or to be obese in our country up until the middle of the 20th century, because we subsisted on a high-fat and high-protein diet, with fewer refined carbs and sugar. The epidemic of degenerative diseases had not yet begun. We had less than 10 percent obesity, and we were a nation of strong people. The diseases obesity causes, such as diabetes and heart disease, were rare.

Until the age of the automobile and the television, our ancestors had plenty of activity that required muscle, and therefore muscle glycogen. Now, as the most sedentary form of our species ever to sit on this planet, we have no muscle size for storing glycogen. Instead, we have muscle *wasting,* even in the young. This is our modern plague. We've gone from *Homo sapiens* to *Homo sedentarius.*

It takes far less muscle to handle a remote and a computer mouse than it does to deal with a saber-toothed tiger, or to cross the Great Plains in a wagon train, or to build a national park and railroad system, or to win two world wars. If you don't have enough muscle, you can't

DR. ROCK REPORTS...
Keep the Food Police
Out of My Kitchen!

Don't tread on me! I want the government off my dinner plate! After 20 years of the "Eating-Wrong Food Pyramid" suggesting that we eat 6 to 11 servings of grain a day, we're left with massive collateral damage. And we're paying for it with unrelenting suffering from a multitude of terminal diseases and trillions of dollars in health care costs for the public now and in the future. Thankfully, the pyramid is gone, and we won't have to look at it on every cereal box and loaf of high-fiber bread any longer. Hopefully it has taught us to be leery of industry-inspired government eating guidelines, because this food folly at our expense was forced on us by the grain and low-fat industries, along with the Physicians Committee for Responsible Medicine, which supported them.

I ask my seminar audiences, "Do you know someone who died of a heart attack?" All hands go up. "Do you know someone who has diabetes?" All hands go up. In the past, if you ate fried eggs and bacon, a steak, or a pork chop instead of high-fiber cereal drowning in soy milk, or some exotic grain from the Andes, you were considered unenlightened, unfeeling, and uneducated, and that's still going on. I ate like that for years, and it almost killed me.

store much glycogen at all. Since insulin is also your fat-storage hormone, once it's unable to make the glycogen delivery, it does another thing it's designed to do. It delivers the excess blood sugar via your liver for conversion to triglycerides that will be circulated in your bloodstream to be burned as energy. However, if you're not moving around all day long, busy and physically active, most of the triglycerides will be shunted to your fat cells for storage, rather than used as fuel.

If your liver and muscle cells are already loaded with plenty of glycogen, these cells become *resistant* to insulin, and more is released. This is a huge problem. Your body is like a warehouse full of boxes from floor to ceiling, with no space for more. Just as the deliveryman is turned away, your muscles and liver refuse to play. Your insulin receptors are saying, "Nope, we're full," to more sugar. Your pancreas senses that you still have high blood sugar, so it pumps out more insulin. This causes the insulin receptor cells to become even more resistant. As the insulin and blood sugar keep building, you're developing a life-threatening situation. Plaque from the thick buildup of sugar in your blood clogs your arteries. You exhaust your pancreas, which keeps pumping out insulin. And at the same time, the insulin works overtime to store this excess sugar as dangerous fat on your body.

Doesn't this make you wonder about all this low-fat food you're encouraged to eat that is usually so high in sugar? Doesn't this force you to question the pervasive recommendations from your doctor for a low-fat, high-carbohydrate diet? Aren't you concerned that current dietary recommendations are still prodding you to eat grains? Aren't our diet "experts" worried about Nutrient Deficiency Disorder, Sedentary Death Syndrome, sarcopenia, metabolic syndrome, diabetes, heart disease, depression, and cancer? These are all carbohydrate-related diseases. The late Weston Price, DDS, a famous dental researcher, spearheaded the only study of its kind, traveling the world before proving conclusively that dental disease, cavities, malformed dental arches, and gum disease are not caused by fat and protein; they're the direct result of a high-sugar, high-carbohydrate, low-fat diet. You can prove this last point to yourself. Drop carbohydrates and sugars from your diet for just a few days and you'll see that your mouth will be cleaner, with less bacterial odor and plaque.

YOUR BODY CAN MAKE CARBOHYDRATES!

There are those who argue that the brain needs glucose for fuel. Therefore, you must provide carbohydrates. Yes, we can provide natural carbohydrates, like those found in vegetables and dairy products. But if the body detects that we are skimping on the vegetables and not getting enough carbohydrates, it creates its glucose in a process called gluconeogenesis. This is a natural process that kicks in automatically to fuel the brain and other organs.

Gluconeogenesis is always accompanied by thermogenesis—the generation of heat in the body as more calories are burned in the process of converting some of the abundant protein you are eating into the carbs you need. The body converts the number of carbs you need without excess. It doesn't overdo carbs the way you do when you say to yourself, "The cupcake was enough; I don't need the icing," but then you eat the icing anyway.

A study in the *Journal of the American College of Nutrition* in which women ages 19 to 22 were put on either a high-protein diet or a high-carbohydrate diet showed the molecular effects of thermogenesis. Women who ate the high-protein diet generated 100 percent more body heat $2\frac{1}{2}$ hours after the meal compared with the carbohydrate eaters. This means they were warmer and burning more calories. As you emphasize whole proteins and the fats they contain in your diet, through thermogenesis you will become a "hottie," too.

CHAPTER **16**

How to Slay the Diabetes Dragon

LOWER YOUR BLOOD SUGAR AND LIVE MUCH BETTER, HEALTHIER, AND LONGER

All the metabolic syndrome diseases—diabetes, heart disease, inflammation, and high blood pressure—are prevalent today because of sugar and grain. Both of these popular foods raise blood sugar. Even whole grains that burn more slowly end up as sugar in your blood. There could be nearly 40 million people with diabetes in the country within 40 years. If habits don't change, this number will include you and your children and most people age 40 and under today. These prospects are bleak! So we are warning you to begin today to think like a person with diabetes!

Lower blood sugar keeps you young. It not only prevents diabetes but also activates anabolism and preserves the attractive lean look of toned muscle. Lower blood sugar triggers the release of human growth hormone and insulin-like growth factor so you can look and feel more youthful. High blood sugar does the opposite. It triggers insulin, as we've already pointed out; shuts down glucagon, your fat-burning hormone; and triggers cortisol, so you begin to break down your muscle. You feel irritable and depressed, become hostile, and crave more sugar even though your body is starving for protein.

Just as you don't guess about your blood pressure, it makes no sense when diabetes is so rampant to guess about your blood glucose levels. At the very least, be sure your physician checks your blood sugar at your yearly physical. Keep your morning or fasting blood sugar in the lower ranges, between 80 and 100, which is the ideal range. Two hours after meals, blood sugar should not be much higher than 140. If you want to check your own blood sugar, you can easily obtain a relatively painless testing kit in just about any drugstore. You might check your blood glucose levels one week every month, every morning before you eat, to see how you are doing. If your fasting blood sugar in the morning before eating is repeatedly over 126, see your doctor immediately to be checked for diabetes. Over a third of those with diabetes in this country are not yet diagnosed. This is a tragedy since diabetes is a very dangerous disease.

GRAIN DAMAGE!

Grain is a nutrient-deficient food. It lacks sufficient quantities of vitamins and minerals to sustain life as your primary food. It's poor in the high biological proteins, particularly the muscle-building amino acids valine, leucine, and isoleucine, as well as the amino acids that help protect against infection, lysine and cysteine. It does not provide the fat or the fat-soluble vitamins you need in readily accessible quantities, nor does it contain the most recently discovered and possibly the greatest fat of them all: conjugated linoleic acid.

Our present dietary guidelines are shaped by a medical tradition that is not adequately attentive to the study of nutrition and the vast body of science that has explored the so-called value of grains versus whole proteins and saturated fats. The guidelines are based on outdated research. The medical mind is so poorly educated in nutrition that we can't look in that direction for answers. It's like asking a plumber to be an electrician. Misconcepts are just trotted out as truth, and you're expected to swallow them—*and you have.* We're far from where we need to be with the new diet guidelines. Vegetables are good, of course, but the emphasis on grains and vegetables and lean and low-fat protein and dairy at the expense of anabolic protein and fat is perpetuating the two silent epidemics of SeDS and nutrient deficiency disorder. You are in line for so many diseases that the list would make your head spin. Doctors can't tell you this. It's up to you to make the appropriate choice for the nutrient advantage and anabolism.

Despite all we're revealing, you may be holding on to the idea that your high-fiber whole grain cereal is keeping you healthy. High fiber is shown by science to be *so hard* on your digestive tract (which was not designed for the coarse quality of whole grains and the gluey quality of refined grains) that you can suffer from gas, bloating, and other discomforts because you're eating it. If it's fiber you're seeking, fresh fruits and vegetables and legumes have plenty of it, in the gentle form that nature designed for our bodies. You'll also find plenty of the right kind of fiber for humans in raw nuts and seeds—no list of ingredients necessary. However, your true laxative is fat! The healthy fats have a laxative effect on some of us—if that's even the right term. High-fat food is designed to move through you effortlessly. Lean and low-fat proteins, in our experience, may clog you since they are devoid of the natural lubrication that ends constipation. Animal fats are the ticket for getting yourself off high fiber and laxatives. The French know to put butter on their steaks from years of experience; we do this, and so can you. From the beginning of time, your colon was designed to work best with the natural lubricants from a high-saturated-fat diet.

THE 72-HOUR OPTION

If you're hooked on carbs, you would be smart to make a small effort to break your addiction. Take advantage of what we call the 72-hour option. Go 2 days without carbohydrates, and then have a carb meal on the third day. You'll love how you slim down on this formula. You'll see pants that were too tight becoming looser very quickly!

One caveat if you want to knock out Nutrient Deficiency Disorder: Do not include any form of refined sugar or sweets in the 72-hour option. You will do best when you enjoy the natural carbs available to you—the yams and potatoes, including their skins (which vastly lower their glycemic rating) and whole grains. This means you can have delicious raisin French toast with fresh blueberry banana compote. Sweet and delicious for breakfast or brunch, this tastes just like dessert. You'll find plenty of recipes in this book to help you keep on eating healthy during your 72-hour carb break. We highly recommend that you follow this processed sugar–free diet for 3 months—completely eliminating all processed sugar as well as flour, which has the same insulin-spiking/fat-storing effect, until you know you're in control of your sugar habit. It won't be hard to cut way back on sugar, because when you eat protein and fat in optimal amounts *you don't crave it.* Imagine that! Your sugar craving is a protein and fat deficiency! You will not have the results you're seeking in fat loss if you keep munching on sugar snacks, or salty treats, or any plastic-covered, 100-year-shelf-life desserts.

It is not our purpose to deny you anything, but rather to educate you to make better choices. To end NDD, you are sooner or later going to have to begin to consider an end to eating sweets and refined and complex carbohydrates. These are energy-robbing foods, since they destroy your nutrient advantage.

Take 3 months and eat whole proteins and fats, plenty of vegetables, and a small quantity of fruit, and make a habit of no longer relying on processed sugars and grains. The rule is that it takes just 30 days to form a new habit, but we want you to extend this experience into a second and then a third month, because the processed sugar and grain habit is so deeply ingrained. You'll continue slimming down and removing the layer of fat from the muscle you're firming. And you'll no longer have a carbohydrate addiction. Once the 90 days are over, you'll be in control. If you want a sweet treat once in a while, you'll be able to

Marilyn's Message...

In 1975, as the very first step in my search for better health, I made the decision to give up sugar completely. I was tired of mood swings and depression and never really having any energy. I was only 31, and I couldn't accept that I wasn't in the best possible health of my life at that age. I went cold turkey after deliberately overeating on doughnuts, which I knew were my absolute worst addiction. I made myself so sick I couldn't look at a doughnut, and from that point on, for 18 years, I never touched sugar. I detested the taste of it.

This worked for me. For some people, it might not work. But at this time in my life, with grandchildren and family gatherings, I always say, "No, thank you. No dessert (or candy)." Because I just don't like it.

indulge and not become lost in the addiction. Some people stop liking sugar completely. We did! You'll be able to regulate the appropriate amount in your diet, when relevant. What is this appropriate amount? We'll pinpoint that for you in the next section.

THE ADA DIET FOR DIABETES

The American Diabetes Association (ADA) has been prescribing a carb-atrocious diet for the carbohydrate-sensitive and endangered population in our country.

According to the ADA, if you have diabetes, you should eat a diet that is 45 to 65 percent carbohydrates. Your protein intake should be 20 percent, and it should be lean, limited as much as possible to fish and chicken. Your fat intake should be around 15 percent.

DR. ROCK REPORTS...

The American Diabetes Association tells those with diabetes to consume 65 percent of their calories from carbs. This is tantamount to telling alcoholics that the best way to end alcoholism is to have a few drinks every day. This current edict is totally out of step with the evidence. Every decade since the 1950s, the US population has increased its sugar consumption, and all the degenerative diseases have risen in tandem, particularly diabetes and heart disease. The Centers for Disease Control and Prevention states that only two-thirds of those with diabetes are counted in official estimates; the real figures are closer to 40 million. Forecasters conclude that the 40 million figure will more than double by 2034. At the same time, the cost of treating people with diabetes will triple, rising from an estimated $113 billion in 2009 to $336 billion in 2034. This staggering figure will most likely bankrupt our country. "We may actually be underestimating what's happening, which is very disturbing," says Elbert Huang, MD, associate director of the Chicago Center for Diabetes Translation Research at the University of Chicago.

Realistically, we don't have a health care system that can handle such a catastrophe of suffering. The greatest danger now is to the millions of innocent people who are heeding the ADA's dietary guidelines and obediently cutting back on the most nutrient-dense whole proteins and fats in favor of the very foods that diabetes patients cannot process: sugars, grains, fruits—essentially all carbohydrates.

I'm one of the people the ADA targets with its high-carbohydrate recommendations. In February 2009, on my 56th birthday, after a period of alarming muscle loss, I was unexpectedly diagnosed with the least common and most dangerous form—late-onset type I diabetes—an autoimmune disorder that destroys the beta cells in the pancreas that produce insulin. Although an anabolic diet had for many years been my focus, 10 years prior to my diagnosis, I began testing three theories: (1) the government's low cholesterol mandate; (2) the vegan diet based on the Cornell-China-Oxford study, stressing soy and a cut in protein to 7 percent with a focus on rice and vegetables; and (3) the raw food movement, which emphasizes eating large quantities of fruit. I'd also taken up long hours of cardio and was studying hatha yoga. Mind you, these were *my personal experiments* to disprove new dietary fads that were, in my opinion, harmful and false. My willingness to leave behind my lifelong philosophy of the anabolic diet and weight-bearing exercise to prove my point backfired: I paid the price. At that time, I was gaunt, yet I was eating constantly, unaware initially that my pancreas no longer produced the insulin to deliver nutrients to my cells. After my shocking diagnosis, I received the prescription for insulin that I would have to take for the rest of my life and a heartbreaking laundry list of what I was now facing: 76 percent greater risk of heart attack; retinopathy, leading to blindness; and potential peripheral neuropathy, leading to amputation. When Marilyn shared her grief with her father, Bernard L. Horecker, PhD, dean of Weill Cornell Graduate School of Medical Sciences, he lamented, "Don has been struck by a most devastating disease." All I knew was that each morning when I injected insulin, a fragile glass bottle and syringe were now all that separated me from premature death.

For nearly 8 months, I was exhausted and depressed. My body put on fat like never before. Suddenly, another catastrophe hit us. A family tragedy struck and reached a culmination that kept us away from home and access to my insulin for long hours. I was deprived of the enormous amount of rest I required and unaware, because I hadn't been warned, that undue stress could kill me. The requirement for daily travel over long distances, followed by sitting for long hours without food and no rest, under the pressure of unbearable stress over a loved-one's woeful troubles, lasted for well over a week. My inability to eat regularly, rest, and take my insulin as required drove my blood sugar to life-threatening levels. As everything bad that could happen spun out of control, my blood was not liquid like blood, but thick like mud, and this disastrous condition stopped my heart. My 76 percent greater risk of heart attack became my reality.

It was God's blessing that I didn't have a stroke and that I didn't just drop dead. In fact, it still amazes me that I didn't even know I'd had a heart attack. Because of nerve degeneration, some people with diabetes feel no pain in the chest during a heart attack. What I did feel was terrible pain in my lower back and an overwhelming feeling of malaise. I didn't tell Marilyn. She was grieving too much over the lack of justice we'd witnessed. I drove Marilyn home for an hour through a vicious thunderstorm. The moment we were home, I injected my insulin and went straight to bed. She asked me if I was all right, and I said, "I'm just exhausted," but a few hours later, in a state of total alarm, she was driving me at top speed to the hospital. Fast-forward through a series of emergency events I don't even want to think about, and the ER physician is rushing into my room, where Marilyn, in a state of shock and anxiety, is holding my hand. I've been checked in as a diabetic; I'm now being rushed to cardiology. As the ER team works to move me, the ER physician says, "Dr. Schnell, you've had a serious heart attack."

(continued)

The diagnosis was cardiomyopathy and congestive heart failure with a 32 percent ejection fraction, meaning I had only 32 percent of the normal capacity to pump incoming blood out of my heart. I was soon to learn that, medically, this combination of symptoms of cardiovascular disease is considered irreversible and deteriorating. The standard procedure to try stents didn't compute because there were no blockages in my arteries. I was discharged 6 days later with a warning not to lift weights and to stay on the ADA diet for diabetics; the endocrinologist tripled my insulin. Doctors warned me that I could have a second heart attack at any time that I would not survive. They told me that I could live another 5 years at the most. I couldn't share all this with Marilyn. I didn't have the heart to tell her.

At that point, I made the resolution of my life. I would stack the cards against the Grim Reaper. I consulted with one of the top board-certified cardiologists in Florida, Ariel Soffer, MD, who duplicated the test results from my hospitalization. Then, I explained my own plan of exercise, supplements, and diet so that he could monitor my results. My research on how diabetes was treated prior to insulin and prior to the huge increase in sugar consumption in this country showed that removing carbs from the diet was the most successful treatment because carbs always spike blood sugar. Coupled with this, my theory was that if I could slowly and systematically increase my strength with carefully measured increases in weights over time, my heart strength would have to accommodate. The added muscle I planned to build would naturally burn excess sugar out of my blood for fuel. I would eat whole proteins and fats, which don't spike blood sugar and say no to all simple sugars, adding only a controlled amount of nonstarchy complex carbs. With Marilyn at my side, doing everything I did at her level of strength, we worked on a well-thought-out weight-bearing exercise and nearly carb-free anabolic regimen. My body toned up and looked muscular. Marilyn looked sexy and gorgeous. Both of us were rejuvenating. We were thriving on the diet Marilyn designed for this book and our routine of progressive resistance training.

Next, Dr. Soffer checked my blood sugar less than 6 months into this regimen. It had dropped from the original diagnosis of 11.9 (1 percentage point from death) to 6.2, which means that I was just barely diabetic.

In March 2011, Dr. Soffer retested my heart. To my surprise, immediately after the results came back from the lab, he ran the test again. I had confidently already shared with him on the basis of how I felt that he would see better results. Dr. Soffer called Marilyn and me to his office with the second set of test results in his hands. "Rock," he said, "I can't explain what I'm seeing. Your ejection fraction has risen from 32 to 58 percent. As far as I'm concerned, miraculously, you're in the normal range. But I have to tell you, man, this doesn't happen. It's not in the medical textbooks. From congestive heart failure and cardiomyopathy, all data says what you've done is impossible."

It was not impossible. I accomplished this on the basic principles of anabolism that Marilyn and I share in this book. There was, however, one other factor: We never gave up our faith. Our love for each other and our determination to be together was handed over to God the moment we hit this crisis. And we never lost the conviction that our prayers would most mercifully be answered.

There is no one-size-fits-all solution to diabetes. And no one should try to duplicate what I did without consulting with a doctor, just as I did. However, the majority of people with diabetes are not type 1, as I am. They are making insulin, as I couldn't, but their cells are *insulin resistant,* meaning they have massive amounts of sugar in their blood, creating the collateral damage of diabetes that I've discussed. The best solution for too much sugar in your blood (as a type 2 diabetic or prediabetic) may *not* be to keep adding insulin. It may be to cut down on sugar and carbs. However, there is a huge industry of insulin producers whose stockholders want to sell their product and who give millions to the American Diabetes Association. Diabetes is a high-profit business.

Medical science knows that the body of a diabetic cannot process carbohydrates or sugar. Prescribing insulin is an effort to help them process high blood sugar. But does it? Isn't it common sense that if you have this condition of high blood sugar with insulin resistance, meaning your cells won't absorb it, that you shouldn't keep adding more sugar to your blood? Do you put out a fire by adding gasoline? Yet in the "Control Your Diabetes for Life, the Diabetes Food Guide Pyramid," created by the American Diabetes Association, you will see the recommendation that the basis of a diabetic's diet should include six or more servings of grains and starches, plus two to four servings of fruit! *We're talking high blood sugar city!*

I think more research should be done on the diabetes diet. Perhaps the solution is simply to manage carbohydrates by cutting them back in favor of foods that don't spike insulin, such as whole proteins and fats. They might also recommend weight-bearing exercise to develop active muscle tissue that burns blood sugar for fuel. It appears that the American Diabetes Association and their sister organization, the American Dietetic Association, are inadvertently providing the insulin industry with lifelong clients and the immense profits created from the production and sale of insulin and other blood sugar–controlling drugs.

PART FOUR

The Myths
That Kill

CHAPTER **17**

Why Your Fear of Cholesterol Is Dangerous to Your Health

NEW THINKING ABOUT AN OLD DEMON

I n 1953, in *Journal of the Mount Sinai Hospital, New York,* physiologist Ancel Keys, PhD, published a paper that challenged the US government's policy on heart disease as being too limited. His viewpoint also posed a challenge to the health policies of that decade, given that the government's prime focus was on the treatment and prevention of infectious diseases. Heart disease was being treated with costly drugs and surgeries, but very little was being done to prevent it. As infectious diseases were on the decline, heart disease was on the rise. Dr. Keys compared the United States with Italy, showing that four times the number of Americans died from heart attacks than Italians. He said that America should take an aggressive stand toward preventing this growing threat. He challenged us to set a hard-hitting prevention agenda, as was being done in other countries. And he already had his eye on how: Attack the high-fat diet.

Dr. Keys was formulating his cholesterol-lipid hypothesis, a theory based on his study of fat consumption and coronary heart disease rates, which was the precursor to his famous Seven Countries Study. This was 1953, and he studied 22 countries but chose to report on only six countries. So we'll call this the Six Countries Study of 1953. The time was right for him, although it's highly debatable that this was *our* "lucky" moment as a population. We say this because this one step was the turning point that ushered in the low-fat era. The essential nutrient saturated fat, which we'd always eaten in abundance in the form of whole proteins from meat and dairy, began to take its fall.

Dr. Keys said he discovered in the six countries he studied that greater saturated fat consumption in men ages 55 to 59 correlated to higher incidence of heart disease in that population. The trend was unmistakable, according to Dr. Keys. There was just one little problem. Dr. Keys talked about only six countries: Australia, Canada, Italy, Japan, the United Kingdom, and the United States. However, his graphs revealed that he had actually studied 22 countries. Where were the results from the other 16 countries? We want to know, because this little study had the effect of sending both of our dads into the kitchen (where we used to enjoy breakfasts of bacon and eggs) to rustle up boring bowls of oatmeal or pour cornflakes out of a box instead. And then we had to eat them with *skim milk!* To this day, we have memories of how the children of that era, like us, moaned about the loss of whole milk, eggs, and bacon.

So, here's what happened. Dr. Keys selected only the six countries that fit nicely into his bias toward his preconceived conclusion. If all the countries were left on the graph, there was no conclusion to be drawn. There was no pattern among the 22 countries showing a correlation between the consumption of saturated fat and heart disease. The results were all over the map; it looked like someone had discharged a shotgun at the graph. By placing the six countries on their own graph, however, Dr. Keys claimed to be *proving* that saturated fat was the cause of heart disease.

He was trying to duplicate a perfect upward arc of his graph to match a graph of mortality in men from heart disease in these six countries. To accomplish that, he needed Australia to fall in line right next to Canada. He called his version of how these six countries lined up in a perfect upward trajectory "The Upward Curve of Doom." Sure enough, it showed that fat and cholesterol consumption in these six countries perfectly correlated to increasing levels of heart disease.

"It is now acknowledged that the original studies purporting to show a linear relation between cholesterol intake and coronary heart disease may have contained fundamental study design flaws," wrote Peter J. Jones, PhD, in a 2009 review of studies on dietary cholesterol, egg consumption, and cardiovascular disease in the *International Journal of Clinical Practice*. Dr. Jones is a professor of food science and nutrition at the University of Manitoba's Richardson Centre for Functional Foods and Nutraceuticals.

Dr. Keys's first big moment for his Six Countries Study came in 1955, when he presented it to the World Health Organization. The international body of scientists didn't get to see the 22-country graph, but, even so, they were relatively unimpressed by the six-country graph he showed. It wasn't conclusive to them. The results appeared too simplistic. It is perhaps for this reason that Dr. Keys's original research document of this study is not anywhere on the Internet.

Dr. Keys pushed forward with a passion. A man on a mission, he was working on a preconceived conclusion that he wished to solidify. He had made the decision that saturated fat and cholesterol were the cause of heart disease. To support his personal viewpoint, he didn't report about the countries where people eat *a lot* of fat but suffer from very little heart disease. He also failed to mention that he found countries where people *don't* eat a lot of fat and yet still have high levels of heart disease.

The first dissent, which would herald a 6-decade-long argument over Dr. Keys's hypothesis, began to rumble from fellow scientists. Jacob Yerushalmy, PhD, founder of the biostatistics graduate program at the University of California, Berkeley, questioned why Dr. Keys had not included data for all countries. Why wasn't it called the 22 Countries Study? When all 22 countries were analyzed on one graph as they initially appeared, Dr. Keys's hypothesis evaporated faster than a drop of water in a hot skillet.

Right after Dr. Yerushalmy's protest of Dr. Keys's findings, Dr. Keys began a second study in 1958, which would be called the Seven Countries Study. It was finished in 1964 but not published until 1970.

Other researchers saw through the myth. In Volume 2 of *Diet, Blood Cholesterol, and Coronary Heart Disease: A Critical Review of the Literature,* Russell L. Smith, PhD, and Edward R. Pinckney, MD, concluded that the Keys study was flawed by such a "massive set of inconsistencies and contradictions" that it could not "be taken seriously by the objective and critical scientist." In one example, Drs. Smith and Pinckney pointed out that the mortality rate in Finland was 24 times that of Mexico, even though fat consumption in both countries was identical. How then could Dr. Keys insist that dietary fat causes heart disease? So, actually, Dr. Keys had failed as a scientist. His work simply didn't stand up to the rigors demanded by science itself. In fact, many other scientists would say that Dr. Keys's data suggested the opposite of his conclusions.

In the book *Fat and Cholesterol Are Good for You,* Uffe Ravnskov, MD, PhD, meticulously describes the long-standing body of research that disproves Dr. Keys's hypothesis. Despite Dr. Ravnskov's abundance of peer-reviewed research and the countless other books and scientific publications that discredit Dr. Keys's findings, Dr. Keys succeeded in blaming heart disease on saturated fat and cholesterol and changed the course of the dietary habits in our country from the 1950s until today. These findings created a groundswell of fear that the foods we'd been eating for as long as we could remember would give us heart disease. Suddenly, old-fashioned butter was the killer demon, and trans fat–laden margarine was the angel that would save us. Daily were the reminders making us feel guilty if we didn't agree that processed and high-sugar cereals were better for us than our traditional bacon-and-eggs breakfast. Over time, steak slowly became unfashionable, no longer coveted as the American food that brought us strength and beauty. It was a guilty pleasure at best. And our fear led to confusion over the traditional Fourth of July barbecue menu. Were we really supposed to begin substituting tofu dogs and burgers on the grill?

This 1953 study drew so much support from so many in medicine and in the food and pharmaceutical industries, it single-handedly launched the cults of low-fat, low-cholesterol, and high-soy diets in our country. Scientists who have spoken out vociferously over the past 60 years maintain that the Keys study was deceptive. Millions of people have died needlessly because this one falsified study triggered a change in dietary habits that resulted in today's widespread health epidemics of obesity, heart disease, cancer, and diabetes.

STILL NOT CONVINCED? CHECK OUT THE MANY INCONSISTENCIES

Today, our government is still pushing the low-fat, low-cholesterol diet in our schools, in the military, to those with diabetes, and to the media and the general population. This is happening in the face of published studies clearly showing that fat and cholesterol are not to be feared, such as:

• In populations of the elderly, the amount of saturated fat and cholesterol in the diet has *nothing* to do with the level of heart disease. Those with high cholesterol often have very little atherosclerosis and live a long time, and those with low cholesterol often die from high levels of atherosclerosis.

• There is no dispute whatsoever that women have slightly higher cholesterol than men, but they have a lower incidence of atherosclerosis, which is perhaps partly due to hormones.

• An analysis of studies at the National Heart, Lung, and Blood Institute revealed a shocking conclusion: Women with low cholesterol die more often from heart disease than women with high cholesterol.

• Consider this study published in 1960: In more than 1,000 autopsies of Americans and Japanese (Jamaican and Indian subjects were studied as well), the aorta—the main artery of the body—was graded for signs of atherosclerosis. The average level of blood cholesterol for Americans at that time was 220; for Japanese it was only 150. Yet, contrary to Dr. Keys's hypothesis, lower cholesterol apparently didn't protect the Japanese subjects from atherosclerosis. Their arteries were almost as full of plaque as the arteries of the Americans.

• More recently, in 2001, the *British Medical Journal* reported a systematic review of 27 randomized clinical trials with a total of 3,902 people who reduced or modified their dietary fat intake for at least 6 months, looking at the effect this had on cardiovascular disease and cardiovascular deaths. The effect was almost negligible: Total mortality decreased a mere 2 percent.

• A Hawaiian study of 3,572 subjects, reported in the British journal *Lancet* in 2001, showed an increased mortality in elderly people with low serum cholesterol.

• A whole set of studies from peer-reviewed journals shows that consuming one to seven eggs per week does not increase the risk of dying from cardiovascular disease or stroke in men or women. Better yet, there was a trend for men with higher egg consumption to have an even lower rate of stroke.

• In 1995, in the *American Journal of Clinical Nutrition,* researchers reviewed trends in heart disease and stroke mortality in Spain from 1966 to 1990. The findings showed that since 1976, there had been a decrease in cardiovascular disease deaths in Spanish men and women. During this same time, the national intake of meat, dairy, fish, and fruit increased. As the population increased its consumption of these products, there was a decrease in the consumption of sugar, carbohydrates, and olive oil. How could this be if the Ancel Keys cholesterol-lipid hypothesis were true? This would come to be known as the Spanish paradox.

• You are probably also aware of the French paradox, which has shown in countless studies that eating butter, an abundance of high-fat cheeses, and plenty of meat does not cause high levels of heart disease in France. Obesity is rare in France.

DON'T IGNORE THE LIFESAVER CALLED VITAMIN E

Richard A. Passwater, PhD, has been one of America's leading nutrition-focused biochemists since 1959. He is credited with legitimizing megavitamin therapy through 46 books on nutrition, including the bestseller

Supernutrition: Megavitamin Revolution. He says, "The discredited hypothesis that eating cholesterol increases the risk of heart disease was based on imperfect circumstantial evidence." Dr. Passwater was so adamant about his beliefs that he said he would donate the proceeds from his book *Supernutrition for Healthy Hearts* to the American Heart Association if anyone could prove that eating cholesterol causes heart disease. There were no takers. No one ever stepped forward.

Included in Dr. Passwater's arsenal of dissenting data was research on vitamin E, which supported the work of the Shute brothers (see Chapter 8). Dr. Passwater pointed directly to research in the *American Journal of Clinical Nutrition* showing that the single most reliable risk factor for heart disease is vitamin E deficiency. Dr. Passwater's research on cardiovascular health and vitamin E was published in *Prevention* magazine in 1971, when he was the first to inform the public of research on antioxidants and free radicals. In 1976, *Prevention* published more of Dr. Passwater's research, this time showing that long-term consumers of vitamin E had less than half the heart disease risk of typical Americans of the same sex and age who did not take the vitamin.

Unfortunately, government and medical experts failed to give a fair hearing to these studies. Instead, the public remained uninformed and therefore unwilling to abandon the anti-saturated-fat and anticholesterol chorus in favor of vitamin E supplementation. As a result, you've been watching your fat intake like a hawk. You've been eating sugar and other carbohydrates in an effort to quell your hunger pangs. You've probably developed a carbohydrate addiction. Do you ever find yourself, hours after your low-fat dinner, in your pajamas, polishing off ice cream or leftover birthday cake in the kitchen?

CHAPTER 18

Billions of Dollars Fail to Prove the Cholesterol-Lipid Hypothesis

MISINFORMATION IS HIDING THE TRUTH ABOUT WHAT'S REALLY CAUSING HEART DISEASE.

Do you believe in unicorns? Not likely; and by the end of this section, it's not likely you'll still believe that bread is better for you than butter. In fact, you may even come to realize that the low-fat cure for heart disease was a big fat mistake.

Although Ancel Keys was not a cardiovascular specialist, but rather a physiologist, he promoted the cholesterol-lipid hypothesis very successfully. He was so adept at promoting himself and his research work that he even appeared on the cover of *Time* magazine on January 13, 1961. The Keys theory connecting cholesterol to heart disease spread to Australia, Canada, the British Isles, and Finland, as the National Institutes of Health and the FDA sent out missionaries of the hypothesis to convert others. Sadly, this would lead to a huge political and economic commitment by the United States government to ensure that plenty of research would be funded to prove this hypothesis, upon which our entire eating culture would come to be based.

The story reads like a thriller, as proponents of Dr. Keys from the government, medicine, and the low-fat, grain, and dairy industries tried desperately to drown out the voices of cardiologists and scientists who criticized the 1953 Keys study as a sham. The uproar from science was controlled so that the public knew nothing about it. Meanwhile, the Keys study gave birth to an entirely new low-fat industry, new dietary guidelines, and greater government control over our food supply.

Dissent came swiftly. In 1964, just a few years after Dr. Keys's *Time* cover, the world-famous heart surgeon Michael DeBakey, MD, and his team of colleagues proved that the cholesterol-lipid hypothesis was actually false. Their study looked closely at 1,700 surgical patients and found that there was no correlation between the patients' blood cholesterol levels and the extent of coronary heart disease. This landmark study, reported in the *Journal of the American Medical Association,* found that about 50 percent of people hospitalized for heart attacks or undergoing coronary artery bypass surgery had normal cholesterol levels. Yet it didn't appear to make a single dent in Dr. Keys's unproven hypothesis that damned saturated fat. The DeBakey study was virtually ignored in the news because the media believed in unicorns.

A CHANGE OF HEART

Cardiologist Stephen Sinatra, MD, who founded the New England Heart Center, says he was once a "cholesterol choirboy" who gave lectures on behalf of Merck and Pfizer, makers of cholesterol-lowering statin medications. But years of clinical practice turned Dr. Sinatra from cheerleader to critic. He says he changed his mind about cholesterol because he could not ignore the following observations:

1. Many patients with low cholesterol will go on to develop heart disease.

2. In many patients with cholesterol above 280, angiograms show normal coronary arteries. They don't have heart disease.

3. Population studies discredit cholesterol as a cause of heart disease. For example, the French have the highest cholesterol levels in Europe—234 back in 1994—and they also have the lowest incidence of heart disease.

4. Half of all heart attacks occur in people who have normal total cholesterol.

SPEAKING OUT CAN BE COSTLY

Another respected medical doctor who refused to believe the alleged harm from saturated fat and cholesterol is heart-bypass pioneer Dwight C. Lundell, MD. A former physician for NASA astronauts, he became a founding partner of the Lutheran Heart Hospital (now Banner Heart Hospital) in Mesa, Arizona—the second largest heart hospital in the United States. This cardiologist performed more than 5,000 open-heart surgeries in his 30-plus-year career. He wrote about his position on high cholesterol in his book *The Great Cholesterol Lie*, in which he argued that the dangers to the heart from saturated fat and cholesterol had no scientific or physiological validity and caused an innocent population to be put at risk. For simply writing his medical opinion in a book that the mainstream could access in his effort to stem the harmful tide he saw coming in American heart health, Dr. Lundell became a target of Quackwatch, a group founded by Stephen Barrett, MD, that attacks doctors who embrace nutritional and naturopathic cures. Quackwatch does great damage to the public in its dedication to serving pharmaceutical interests and the medical monopoly. For providing solid arguments that discredited the Ancel Keys low-fat movement, Dr. Lundell found himself harassed and personally and professionally scrutinized by the National Council Against Health Fraud, which is affiliated with Dr. Barrett and Quackwatch.

However, Dr. Barrett—the leading voice against chiropractic and other forms of alternative medicine—was actually exposed as a fraud himself, misrepresenting himself as a medical and legal expert although he is not a licensed physician and holds no legal degree. In the Superior Court of Los Angeles County (case number BC245271), Judge Haley J. Fromholz ruled against Dr. Barrett and the National Council Against Health Fraud on April 22, 2003. Judge Fromholz found Dr. Barrett and his partner, Wallace I. Sampson, MD, to be misrepresenting their credentials and using witnesses who were unqualified and without adequate knowledge to prove their case. In addition, he found that they were paid by the National Council Against Health Fraud specifically to win cases that enrich the council's litigation funds. Since Dr. Barrett was a board member of the National Council Against Health Fraud, he's enriched by every case he wins. During the trial, his license had not been current for 7 years, and the judge found him to be misrepresenting his credentials and expertise.

You may think this is a rarity, but it is not. For years, this organization has done great damage in its attacks against alternative health writers and the professions of chiropractic, homeopathy, and many other alternative practices. But this problem is not limited to private organizations that represent themselves as public servants. There are plenty of attack dogs in the government who take on whistle-blowers.

On July 14, 2012, the *New York Times* reported that the FDA spied on e-mails its own scientists sent to congress members, journalists, labor officials, and even the president. Let's be clear: According to the *Times* article, the FDA used spy software in retaliation against government scientists who were blowing the whistle on secret methods the agency uses to hide the danger of certain medical devices from the public. Make no mistake. This is not uncommon. This is a clear example of politics and profits denying you your right to be healthy.

The good news is that Dr. Lundell has not been deterred in his fight to tell the true story. He called attention to a study regarding saturated fats and heart disease in an article published in the *American Journal of Clinical Nutrition* on January 13, 2010. He said the study of 347,747 subjects found that there was no association between the intake of saturated fat and heart disease or stroke.

Is your doctor informed about this? We hope so. But we doubt it. Lamentably, none of this vital information has reached our decision makers. As recently as July 2012, direct from the White House came the urging that our troops be served low-fat food choices. The suggestion was even made to the troops to set the example for the public by consuming and eating low-fat foods. What a vicious cycle! This shows how entrenched this information has become. Leading medical journals are saying there is no correlation, but the policy makers just keep marching to the beat of an outdated drummer. It's a wave of untruth sweeping the facts out of its path. But the inconvenient truth is that the more low-fat foods we eat, the more our waistlines expand, and what follows is the continuous rise in the epidemics of obesity, heart disease, diabetes, and cancer. Before the low-fat era, the number of obese people in our country had been hovering below 15 percent for decades. Now, on low-fat diets, we're moving up toward 35 percent.

In an interview with Doctor Watch, a blog set up by doctors to counteract the claims of Quackwatch, Dr. Lundell said, "In spite of the fact that there was no initial evidence to support the low-fat theory in the first place, the diet continues to be the focus of the government, the medical establishment, and almost every food manufacturer in this country. The American public is screaming for change. And, instead of looking closely at the low-fat theory and its results on our health—more incidences of heart disease and obesity—those in power ignorantly continue lowering the fat content of our food supply. The lower it gets, the fatter we become. And heart disease is out of control."

MAYBE IT'S YOUR FRIES AND PIES

We have only scratched the surface in this chapter, but our conclusion, based on mountains of research, is that there is no legitimate scientific support for the idea that cholesterol and saturated fat in animal proteins will clog your arteries and cause heart disease. In fact, according to a report in the medical journal *Lancet* in 1994, only about 26 percent of the fat in artery clogs is saturated fat; the rest is primarily polyunsaturated fat.

This should shock you! What we're talking about here is the fat in your fries and pies, not in your steak and burgers. Television experts and the general dietetic and medical population are almost always touting the dangerous misinformation that these polyunsaturated fats are preferable fats.

LOW-FAT-DIET MYTH BUSTING

Doctors, government, and nutrition experts will often raise the argument that the low-carbohydrate diet has not been sufficiently tested. This is simply not true. Plenty of research gives us evidence that there's no benefit from a low-fat diet, but there is probable harm.

But first, just to give you an example of how much you have to wade through to find the real scoop on this issue, let's review one study that comes up frequently to show you just how sloppy the research on low-fat diets has been. We think this one example may blow your mind.

The Women's Health Initiative was a huge 8-year government study that began recruiting volunteers in 1993 and cost American taxpayers over a quarter of a billion dollars. More than 48,000 healthy women, average age 62, participated to find out whether a low-fat diet could prevent cancer and heart disease. This study, however, failed to test the saturated fat–heart connection in so many ways that it's hard to believe. It found that a low-fat diet had no effect on preventing breast cancer in the 8 years of the study. When it came time to assess how a low-fat diet affected heart disease, the researchers concluded that reduced fat intake did not significantly reduce the risk of heart disease or stroke. Although the test group cut fat to 29 percent of calories, researchers rationalized too late that it should have been cut to 20 percent.

The second problem was that no type of fat was specified. The women could eat whatever type of fat they preferred, so no researcher really knew what the participants were eating. This entire expensive study on saturated fat and heart disease *did not test specifically for saturated fat!* Compared with the test group of about half the women in the study who were put on a high-fiber grain, fruit, and vegetable diet, the low-fat group showed no reduction in their risk of disease. So, the study indicated that the low-fat diet was not the magic bullet against cancer and heart disease that was hoped for.

The point we're making is that even when the research fails to prove *anything,* the low-fat gospel is so entrenched that the knee-jerk response is to robotically keep repeating it as if they're trumpeting success and validation.

Now, let's consider data from the highly touted Nurses' Health Study by Harvard University researchers and the Health Professionals Follow-Up Study. Both of these studies found no link between overall percentages of calories from fat and any dietary fat and heart disease or weight gain.

THE ISRAELI STUDY THAT DESTROYS THE LOW-FAT DIET

In a study published in the *New England Journal of Medicine* on July 17, 2008, scientists, including the famed Meir Stampfer, MD, DrPH, a professor of epidemiology and nutrition at the Harvard School of Public Health, concluded that a low-carb diet and a Mediterranean-style regimen helped people lose more weight than a traditional low-fat diet—nearly 12 pounds versus 7 for the low-fat dieters. This was one of the longest and largest studies to ever compare different weight loss strategies. What's more, the researchers found that the low-carb diet improved cholesterol more than the other two. Some critics had predicted the opposite.

The study is remarkable because it lasted 2 years, much longer than most, and even more so because it was in a totally controlled setting with nearly 85 percent of participants completing the diet study. The research was performed in an isolated nuclear research facility in Israel. The 322 participants got their main meal of the day, lunch, at a central cafeteria.

"The workers can't easily just go out to lunch at a nearby Subway or McDonald's," said Dr. Stampfer, the study's senior author, in an article in the *Washington Post.* In the cafeteria, the appropriate foods for each diet were color-coded: red for low fat, green for Mediterranean, and blue for low carb. For breakfast and dinner, the dieters were counseled on how to stick to their eating plans and were asked to fill out questionnaires on what they ate. The participants were also involved in the same level of exercise.

Things haven't changed, even though this alarm has been sounded repeatedly since the 1960s, when Dr. DeBakey did his research. In 2008, John Tierney, a columnist for the Science section of the *New York Times* asked, "If eating more saturated fat improved the dieters' cholesterol profile (while also enabling them to lose weight even though their calories were not restricted), should the federal government and the American Heart Association stop warning people about saturated fats?" To Tierney's question we add this one: Should these powerful governing and opinion-forming groups continue to be encouraging the low-fat diet?

THE NIH PUSHES THE LOW-CARBOHYDRATE DIET

Some positive news: A study conducted by the National Institutes of Health and published in the *Journal of the American Medical Association* in June 2012 concluded that a low-carbohydrate diet is better for weight loss than a low-fat diet. The study found that participants following the low-carb diet burned about 325 calories a day more than they did on the low-fat diet and experienced these key health benefits: increased HDL cholesterol and lowered triglycerides.

To that list we would suggest that a low-carb diet increases energy, improves muscle tone, improves sexual function, triggers better sleep, and delivers greater strength and mental alertness. What we're talking about is anabolism. We're talking about ending Nutrient Deficiency Disorder as a government-sponsored policy. For our government to *mandate* a low-fat, high-carb diet in our school lunch program and in the cafeterias of our soldiers is dangerous. Without the essential protein— the first food for the human body—to create the treasured anabolic conditions, we're going to realize the worst possible outcome for our future: a catabolic country. These nutrients that our leaders and so-called experts demonize actually provide the following health benefits:

• They keep new cells strong.
• They ensure that hormones are plentiful and in balance.
• They hold the wicked witch cortisol at bay and ensure that the angel glucagon is turned on for fat burning.

- They keep moods high rather than in chronic depression.
- They promote the sharp mind and strong bones that come from the nutrients that accompany protein and saturated fat, such as alpha-lipoic acid and vitamin K.
- They prevent fat storing and obesity, followed by diabetes, heart disease, and cancer.

Do you want these prized anabolic conditions for your children? Or do you want them to suffer in catabolism? Do you want your sons and daughters in the military to be anabolic and grow stronger? Or do you want them weak and depressed? You're going to have to take action on this and communicate what you've learned, because the actions against the anabolic life are so massive and so deeply entrenched in the minds of powerful people, knowingly or unknowingly serving the profit-driven pharmaceutical, grain, sugar, and soy industries, that only by popular demand will this low-fat myth ever die.

A CARDIOLOGIST SPEAKS OUT

In a paper titled "The Diet-Heart Hypothesis: A Critique," published in the March 2004 edition of the *Journal of the American College of Cardiology*, Sylvan Lee Weinberg, MD, past president of the American College of Cardiology, says, "The low-fat 'diet-heart hypothesis' has been controversial for nearly 100 years. The low-fat-high-carbohydrate diet, promulgated vigorously by the National Cholesterol Education Program, National Institutes of Health, and American Heart Association since the Lipid Research Clinics Coronary Primary Prevention Trial in 1984, and earlier by the US Department of Agriculture food pyramid, may well have played an unintended role in the current epidemics of obesity, lipid abnormalities, type 2 diabetes, and metabolic syndromes.

"This diet can no longer be defended by appeal to the authority of prestigious medical organizations or by rejecting clinical experience and a growing medical literature suggesting that the much-maligned low-carbohydrate-high-protein diet may have a salutary effect on the epidemics in question."

CHAPTER **19**

The Famous Framingham Heart Study

HOW IT EMBOLDENED THE "CHOLESTEROL CULT" AND CAUSED THE STATIN SCAM

The Framingham Heart Study, which began in 1948 on a population of just over 5,200 men and women, was the earliest organized research on live human subjects in the search for answers to preventing and treating heart disease and associated risk factors. Framingham is one of the most celebrated works of epidemiology in the history of medicine. Prior to Framingham, most epidemiological research was performed using medical records and death certificates. So Framingham deserves wide acclaim as the first study to include vast numbers of live people as subjects.

An early major achievement of the Framingham Heart Study was the discovery through research that smoking was bad for the heart. It is the late William B. Kannel, MD, director of the study from 1966 to 1979 and principal investigator from 1979 until 1987, who is recognized for bringing these findings to the public's attention. Prior to that time, doctors in white coats (or actors playing doctors) were appearing in magazine commercials and on television saying, "More doctors smoke Camels than any other cigarette."

Framingham also blazed new trails in data collection. Since 1987, researchers in the study have collected the DNA of all participants to store in a data bank that has become a treasure trove for genetic research and analysis. Purely in the depth of data gathered and the intention to shed light on heart disease, this study is momentous. Now in its third generation of participants, the study involves the commitment of the first-generation participants, their children, and grandchildren to undergo a thorough medical history, physical examination, and medical tests, including testing of cholesterol and heart health, every 2 years.

Another Framingham achievement relates to findings on cholesterol and saturated fat, and this is the most important.

Do you believe that eating cholesterol raises cholesterol in your blood? Do you believe that high cholesterol in the blood causes heart disease?

If you do, you can let go of these misconceptions, because Framingham disproved both of them. In the longest running and perhaps most significant study on heart disease, Framingham proved that the intake of cholesterol in the diet had absolutely no correlation with heart disease. Remember that cholesterol is contained in saturated fats.

Hold on to your book (or your digital tablet), because you're about to read something that will shock you: Ancel Keys actually believed exactly what the Framingham study found.

In the *Journal of Nutrition* in May 1956, Dr. Keys wrote: "It is concluded that in adult men the serum cholesterol level is essentially independent of the cholesterol intake over the whole range of natural human diets. It is probable that infants, children and women are similar." To make this clear, what Keys is saying is the cholesterol in your diet does not raise the cholesterol in your blood.

THREE POINTS OF LOGIC THAT DEBUNK DR. KEYS'S THEORIES

1. Only animal foods (meat, fish, eggs, and dairy) contain cholesterol. No plant foods, including grains, contain cholesterol.

2. All natural animal foods contain fat—unsaturated and saturated. Some may be lower in saturated fat, but they all contain it.

3. The first two points are inseparable. Cholesterol comes only from an intake of the saturated fat in animal foods.

Dr. Keys said it's not the cholesterol; it's the saturated fat. That's like saying it's not the white; it's the rice. White rice is white. You can't separate the two. If you disqualify one, you must realize that you're disqualifying both.

Dr. Keys's retraction of cholesterol as a culprit shifted his theory to the lipid (fat) hypothesis. But once he freed cholesterol, he couldn't turn around and simply indict saturated fat, because cholesterol and saturated fat come from the same source: animal products. As a physiologist, Dr. Keys didn't get this. Eating a diet high in saturated fat doesn't necessarily mean you will have high cholesterol. And having high cholesterol doesn't necessarily mean you will have heart disease. This may remind you of the well-known French paradox and also the more recently discovered Spanish paradox. The French eat more fat and cholesterol than the population of any other country in the European Union, yet they have the lowest percentage of deaths from coronary heart disease.

The French and Spanish statistics actually aren't paradoxical. There is simply no connection between heart disease and either cholesterol or saturated fat, which are practically one and the same, since they come from the same source. They were both ruled out when cholesterol was ruled out. To repeat this one more time, since you probably heard the opposite 5 minutes ago on television, cholesterol and saturated fat are inseparable and from the same source, so neither one nor the other has any causative effect on heart disease.

If you're still not convinced, since you've been listening for so long to diametrically opposed conclusions, here's what the third director of the Framingham Heart Study, William P. Castelli, MD, said about cholesterol and saturated fat: "In Framingham, Massachusetts, the more saturated fat one ate, the more cholesterol one ate, the *more calories one ate,* the lower the person's serum cholesterol.... We found that the people who ate the most cholesterol, ate the most saturated fat, ate the most calories, weighed the least, and were the most physically active."

LOW CHOLESTEROL CAUSES HEART DISEASE

Now let's look at the most remarkable finding of the Framingham Study, which is a point you will definitely *not* hear the proponents of the Cholesterol Cult discussing on television. Thirty years after the start of the study, researchers asked themselves what had happened. A most shocking discovery was made. The participants whose cholesterol had gone down during those 30 years were actually more likely to die than those whose cholesterol had gone up! "For each 1 [percent] mg/dl drop of cholesterol there was an 11 percent increase in coronary and total mortality," wrote Uffe Ravnskov, MD, PhD, in *Fat and Cholesterol Are Good for You.*

An 11 percent increase in heart disease and death each time there is a 1 percent reduction of cholesterol in our blood?

Framingham proved this!

This gut-wrenching finding has been confirmed repeatedly in other studies as well.

Excuse us! We're going to our kitchen for a moment to fry some eggs in butter. We'll be right back!

High Cholesterol Puts Women on Top

Speaking of eggs, which you may not eat anymore since you've been thrust into the low-fat era, they contain choline, which intensifies the female orgasm. The point here is that every sex hormone that men and women need requires cholesterol as a precursor. That's a fact! You do need to eat for your hormones, although not for your cholesterol readings. This is our experience: Avoiding cholesterol and fat in your diet leaves you with a poor shape to your body, less strength, less fun, and, woefully, less-satisfying sex.

LET MONICA PUT THE CULT TO BED

Following Dr. Keys's establishment of the cholesterol-lipid hypothesis, the World Health Organization conducted a gigantic international study in 1979 on cardiovascular disease called the MONICA Project. MONICA stands for the Multinational MONItoring of Trends and Determinants in CArdiovascular Disease. It included 39 groups of scientists and doctors from 26 countries in North America, Europe, Asia, and Australia, and it focused on every variable that could possibly be of importance in the development of cardiovascular disease, including blood cholesterol. According to MONICA, and much to the surprise of its researchers, there was little if any association between the average level of cholesterol in each country and heart disease mortality.

Why were the researchers surprised? It's like a Keystone Kops film. Everyone is running around looking for what's already found and acting surprised when they find it.

Most cardiologists and other specialists today have no knowledge of MONICA—which isn't surprising at all. It's actually shocking how little time doctors have to update themselves on the "new" science that's been around since 1996, let alone current research. We can switch from 3G to 4G cellphones in a heartbeat. Every doctor has the latest cellphone and iPad, but they don't update their own knowledge. When will they go 4G on the low-fat fiasco?

Fortunately, plenty of medical experts are enlightened on the issue and speak out against the falsity that saturated fat and cholesterol cause heart disease. We've already spoken of Michael R. Eades, MD, and his wife, Mary Dan Eades, MD, authors of *Protein Power*. And world-renowned biochemist Mary G. Enig, PhD, vice president of the Weston A. Price Foundation and author of *Know Your Fats,* says, "The theory is completely and totally wrong."

We've made every effort to show you with an abundance of solid research that the oft-used term *artery-clogging saturated fat* is all part of the vernacular of our times, spoken so frequently that people begin to believe it. At one time, people believed Earth was flat, but we evolved beyond that ridiculous notion. Same goes for the belief that our planet was the center of the universe; now only teenagers feel they are the center of the universe. Some people actually believed that our society would crumble at the start of this millennium. Didn't take long for us to let Y2K go. That's how wrongheaded the idea is that high cholesterol and saturated fat cause heart disease. Surrender to the reality: You've been conditioned to fear cholesterol and saturated fat, and there is not one day that goes by without *something* reminding you to avoid this "bad stuff." It's all over the media, on signs in your supermarket, and on the products in your refrigerator. As wrong as it is, it has taken over your reality. This has brought you sugar and carbs in excess, guilt over your love of a steak, catabolism, impotency, loss of sex drive, depression, aggression, suppression, repression, huge problems with nutrient deficiencies, and not even a remote chance of being anabolic.

Fearing saturated fat and cholesterol, you struggle with a belly that's soft and flabby. You have sarcopenia, diabetes, and heart disease breathing down your neck. But now you've had a chance to review as much as we can include in this book. So much good science has disproved this bogus Keys theory that the subject is worthy of a library full of books.

The basis of a scientific law is that it is a phenomenon of nature that has been proved to occur whenever certain conditions exist or are met. The law of gravity is the same in Paris as it is in Mexico City. Either animal fat raises cholesterol everywhere or it doesn't, and either high cholesterol is the cause of atherosclerosis, heart attacks, and death from heart disease everywhere, in both sexes, and in every age group, or it isn't. AND IT ISN'T! *FRAMINGHAM IS TELLING YOU THIS. MONICA IS TELLING YOU THIS.* Therefore, you're now free from membership or enslavement in the Cholesterol Cult. Sound science has deprogrammed you.

The greatest benefit from this bogus cholesterol theory has been to the manufacturers of margarine, vegetable oils, fat-free and low- or no-cholesterol foods, and, of course, to the grain, soy, sugar, and pharmaceutical industries. If someone serves you one of the butter substitutes, quickly say, "Gee, I can't believe you're not giving me butter."

GOOD AND BAD CHOLESTEROL?

This final piece of dogma of the Cholesterol Cult that we must help you clear out of your mind brings back the unicorn. For too long you've been saddled with the delusion that there are actually such things as good and bad cholesterol. The correct understanding of your body's physiology can completely eradicate this myth and your misunderstanding. Your body produces cholesterol. Cholesterol just *is*. There is nothing that has shown that there are such things as good or bad cholesterol. This is an artificial labeling by misinformed, misguided, medical cultists. The fact is each form of cholesterol serves a vital function in your body.

Your body makes blood, lymph, and cholesterol among all the other substances you need it to make. It makes cholesterol because it knows how necessary this substance is for survival, and it wants to ensure there is always some cholesterol present, in case you don't eat any. From the beginning of time, humans ate plenty. It was all we often had for sustenance from the animals we hunted. Much of the cholesterol your body produces is made in your liver, and the cholesterol you eat is transported to your liver for processing, but the amount you eat, no matter how great, will only cause your cholesterol levels to fluctuate upward or downward a certain percent. The body keeps cholesterol in homeostasis for your needs. From the liver, endogenous and/or exogenous cholesterol are transported by LDL and shuttled to every cell in your body. Why? Because cholesterol is found in the membranes and organelles of every cell in your body! It maintains the integrity of your cell membrane and helps to slightly immobilize the outer surface of the membrane and make it less permeable to very small water-soluble nutrients that could otherwise pass through more easily. It also keeps your cell membrane fluid but not mushy. Cholesterol also facilitates cell signaling, so that cells can communicate and you can function as a human rather than a blob of cells.

Now LDL becomes more easily understood. It's loaded with cholesterol because it has to deliver cholesterol from your liver to where it is urgently needed to repair leaks in the cells or fissures in the arteries. After learning about vitamin C and collagen deficiencies (see Chapter 9), you now realize that you're going to have plenty of fissures in your arteries if your vitamin C level falls below the daily recommended intake of 60 to 75 milligrams. We believe that in people with a vitamin C, vitamin D, or collagen deficiency, cholesterol is forced to play the emergency role of patching the weak areas in cells and tissues. So stop worrying about having too much cholesterol! Whatever cholesterol the body doesn't use in its many tasks for repair and building of your brain cells, hormones, and neurotransmitters, among other things, is picked up and shuttled back to the liver via HDL. So you can visualize HDL and LDL as a railway system, a monorail, or a subway. They are transporters, moving up and down the tracks in your body, delivering and picking up cholesterol. Since LDL moves the cholesterol out and delivers it to where it is needed, and HDL only brings back the excess, you get the picture that there is no negative or positive with either of these. They are just doing what they're designed to do.

Now the fairy tale you've been told over and over again is that LDL is the *bad* cholesterol, and HDL is the *good* cholesterol. This demonizing of a perfectly natural (and rather miraculous) biological process in your body is a classic failure of modern medicine—out of step with its own science. What you are told is a misrepresentation of fact and physiology that convinces you to take a drug to "protect" you, when, in fact, that drug will do the opposite: *It will give you a disease.*

THE STATIN SCAM

Dr. Ravnskov's decades of research caution that pregnant women on statins bear children with birth defects 38 percent of the time, but often pregnant women are put on statins with no warning of this risk. While the *Journal of Obstetrics and Gynaecology Canada* maintains that there is no evidence of this, the nonprofit organization March of Dimes has expressed concern about the dangers to infants when pregnant women are taking statin drugs.

According to Ray Moynihan and Alan Cassels in their book *Selling Sickness,* the majority of "health experts" who created the new cholesterol guidelines in the United States have multiple financial ties to the pharmaceutical firms that make statin drugs. In fact, one of these so-called experts had financial ties to all 10 drug companies. Clearly, this is a conflict of interest and unacceptable.

K. L. Carlson, a former sales rep for statin drugs and the author of *Diary of a Legal Drug Dealer,* has turned whistle-blower on the pharmaceutical industry. She has much to say about the huge amounts of money doctors are paid to push the drugs. The more influential a doctor is, the greater amounts he or she receives. In just one example, as reported in the *Wall Street Journal,* Eli Lilly paid physicians pushing their drugs a whopping $22 million in just the first quarter of 2009.

Carlson shares her great concern about the July 2008 recommendation by the American Academy of Pediatrics that children as young as 2 years of age be tested for high cholesterol and be put on statin drugs based on pharmaceutical companies' guidelines. Stephen R. Daniels, MD, PhD, the lead author of the AAP clinical policy statement, admits to having been a paid consultant to the pharmaceutical companies, according to Carlson.

In their report, "Dangers of Statin Drugs: What You Haven't Been Told about Popular Cholesterol-Lowering Medicines," Mary Enig, PhD, and Sally Fallon write, "Cholesterol is vital to proper neurological function. It plays a key role in the formation of memory and the uptake of hormones to the brain." Cholesterol is the main organic molecule in the brain, constituting over half the dry weight of the cerebral cortex.

Now, what opinions can you form about the idea of giving cholesterol-lowering drugs to children? Is this suggestion worrisome to you? It certainly should be, because it would very probably destroy their chances for proper brain development. In fact, it's a frontal attack on the brain.

Richard A. Passwater, PhD, author of *Supernutrition: Megavitamin Revolution,* and one of the leading specialists in the battle against the Cholesterol Cult, suggests that our medical establishment and the government are wasting time and money on this low-fat diet and low-cholesterol strategy with statins, neither of which have been proven to reduce the death rate from heart disease. He points out that statins have significant side effects on mental cognition, muscle function, and energy. For what benefit? There's no proof that these drugs prevent heart disease.

Look! We've gone through the trauma of heart disease as a couple. We heard all the misinformation from many well-meaning but uninformed doctors who were involved in our case, and we saw this same information being pushed on sick and frightened heart attack victims in hospitals. We were informed that statins always had to be a part of our lives. As for the dietary recommendations, in the hospital we heard,

"Sure! You can eat all the carbs on that tray. The desserts? Of course! Not too much protein! Keep your protein and fat low. Here's margarine, if you want butter. And, most of all, when you return home, do *not* lift any weight!"

We listened, but we resolved to take a different course of action. We started looking for another truth, and we fought this decades-long trend as it loomed in our own personal lives and are now bringing you this lifesaving information. For more than 60 years, right up until the present moment, doctors, dietitians, so-called health specialists from the vegetarian community, and the government have demonized saturated fat and cholesterol and forced the high-carbohydrate, low-fat diet and cholesterol-lowering drugs on the public. Lamentably, after all this indoctrination, we are still a nation facing an epidemic of obesity and diabetes and one where heart disease is still the top killer of both men and women. As millions die unnecessarily, how can they in good conscience continue to cling like barnacles to a false theory that has caused us a tsunami of disease?

The eminent American physician and scientist George V. Mann, MD, former researcher of the Framingham Heart Study and author of the article "Obesity: The Nutritional Spook," in the *American Journal of Public Health,* says, "The diet-heart hypothesis has been repeatedly shown to be wrong, and yet, for complicated reasons of pride, profit and prejudice, the hypothesis continues to be exploited by scientists, fundraising enterprises, food companies and even governmental agencies. The public is being deceived by the greatest health scam of this century, perhaps of any century."

PART FIVE

Outing Sugar

CHAPTER 20

Sweet Deceit

BEWARE OF SUGAR IN ALL ITS DISGUISES.

ugar is bad news. Sugar competes with vitamin C for assimilation into your cells. There goes one of your most powerful antioxidants. Even if your blood sugar reading is on the relatively low end of where it should be, there will still be enough sugar to block your cells' uptake of vitamin C. So forget about having enough vitamin C to create the collagen for firmer, tighter, and younger-looking skin. Even more important, by depriving your cells of vitamin C, sugar depresses your immune system, putting you at risk for infections and disease.

In this chapter and the one that follows, we'll explore just how important it is for you to reduce the sugar that is bombarding your body. We're truly talking about a battle you must do everything in your power to win.

CHILDREN OF THE CORN SYRUP

Have you experienced mood swings? Have you ever witnessed the children's version—a 3-year-old's horrific temper tantrum while standing in the checkout line at the supermarket?

Sugar may be partially to blame. Adrenal exhaustion is caused by all that sugar in baby food, "fruit" juice made from high-fructose corn syrup, fruit leathers, gummy bears, toaster treats, cotton candy, candy bars, granola bars, and sugary cereals.

All carbohydrates, including sugar, *require* B vitamins in order to be converted into energy. But here's the conundrum: The adrenal glands also require B vitamins, and when the adrenals are robbed of B vitamins by excessive carbohydrate consumption, they signal the secretion of cortisol, the stress hormone. The flood of unchecked stress hormones from the adrenal glands can trigger toddler meltdowns as well as anxiety disorders and clinical depression in adults as well as children. According to a study in the *British Medical Journal,* a great number of prescriptions for antidepressants are filled for children.

Another thing happens when the adrenals are deprived of B vitamins: They look to other sources—namely, muscle tissue. If you don't supply your body with B vitamins from eggs, dairy, and meat at meals every 3 to 4 hours, as well as B-complex vitamin supplementation, your muscle is the "meat" your body will turn to in desperation to meet its B vitamin needs. When you drink sweetened iced tea on a hot day and give your child heavily sweetened lemonade, it's all done with love, but it's the result of horrible misdirection. You may as well be playing with a loaded gun.

Doctors themselves are constantly running to the vending machine or snack tray for granola bars and doughnuts. Surgeons are notorious sugar addicts, regularly pounding sodas and candy bars for energy before entering the operating room.

THE BIRTHDAY CAKE SYNDROME

Since the 1960s, one group of medical professionals—the Orthomolecular Physicians, originally led by Linus Pauling, PhD, and Abram Hoffer, MD—has continued to highlight the connection between B vitamin deficiency and mental illness. Sugar causes depression. Consider Columbine, Virginia Tech, and other tragedies involving children. Were these kids eating nutrient-rich diets? Or sugar? We believe they were in severe adrenal shock due to sugar and a lack of B vitamins.

You see the effects of sugar at every birthday party: Kids start out happily eating frosting-slathered birthday cake and end up leaving the party crying uncontrollably. Here's a fact to consider from the World Health Organization: *Depression will be the number two cause of global disease burden by 2020.* The global disease burden measures years of life lost because of premature mortality and time lived in states of less than full health. Depression can also be hard on the heart and could lead to heart disease.

Profit motives are the root of your sugar habit and your child's sugar dependency. It's time to face the catastrophic facts and eliminate sugar.

We've been told over and over again since the 1970s that "fat causes heart attacks." In the '80s, the American Heart Association cookbook featured all kinds of ways to cook without fat. However, a report by Patty W. Siri-Tarino et al. in the January 2010 issue of the *American Journal of Clinical Nutrition* refutes the notion that fat alone causes cardiovascular disease.

Siri-Tarino and her colleagues have affiliations with Children's Hospital Oakland Research Institute; the Center of Excellence for

Marilyn's Message...

In 1975, when I made the decision to begin my research on the effects of food by giving up sugar, my whole life changed. This was the first time I could truly understand how just that one food had been shifting my world steadily in long, downward cycles. I recognized that I was particularly sensitive to sugar. There was no big movement against carbohydrates at that time. We all ate sugary foods, and few thought that we shouldn't until William Dufty's book *Sugar Blues* caught on. I totally understood his breakthrough message. After eating any significant quantity of sugar, I felt my mood swing into depression. (Of course it would! The sugar was destroying my B vitamins.) After I went cold turkey and completely gave up sugar, I never regretted that decision. I ceased to even like the taste of it. And I very much appreciated my ability to maintain energy and greater feelings of well-being.

I lost a layer of fat from much of my body when I left sugar behind, and my body was tighter and firmer. I also lost the premature aging in my skin that, at 31, I was beginning to notice. My skin was clearer, softer, and more radiant, and I looked years younger, just from this one pivotal step. We must always remember that sugar and collagen enter the cells through the same receptors, and when we give up sugar, we are no longer prone to wrinkles! I was only 31, but within just a few months, I looked and felt better than I did at 21, when I was eating sugar.

Nutritional Genomics at the University of California, Davis; and the departments of nutrition and epidemiology at the Harvard School of Public Health. The bottom line of their study is that in order to lower our risk of cardiovascular disease, we should limit our intake of refined carbohydrates. First and foremost, that would be sugar

In addition, Meir Stampfer, MD, DrPH, of the Harvard School of Public Health, says in a *Scientific American* article that the old way of thinking that high cholesterol is a great predictor of risk could be problematic. Dr. Stampfer coauthored a study in the *New England Journal of Medicine* in 2008 that followed 322 moderately obese individuals for 2 years as they adopted one of three diets.

- A low-fat, calorie-restricted diet based on American Heart Association guidelines

- A Mediterranean, calorie-restricted diet rich in vegetables and low in red meat

- A low-carbohydrate, non-calorie-restricted diet.

Dr. Stampfer's study found that the people who ate the low-carb diet and the most saturated fat ended up with the healthiest ratio of HDL to LDL cholesterol, and they also lost twice as much weight as the other groups.

These luminaries in science have underscored the flawed cholesterol-lipid hypothesis that has so many people around the world believing that saturated fat causes obesity, diabetes, and heart disease. Here's our breakthrough: These experts blame these epidemics on sugar and refined carbohydrates. Dr. Stampfer from Harvard is one of the leading epidemiologists in the world. David Ludwig, MD, PhD, is the founder of the Optimal Weight for Life Program in Boston. Robert Lustig, MD, a pediatric endocrinologist at the University of California, San Francisco's School of Medicine, is the leading expert in childhood obesity. In his lectures, he calls sugar a "poison," a "toxin," and an "evil."

Despite all the research evidence and the expert testimony of these scientists, the USDA's Center for Nutrition Policy and Promotion chose to ignore this new thinking on fats and carbohydrates in the 2010 federal Dietary Guidelines for Americans, which are updated every 5 years, in favor of a "short and simple" message. The deputy director of that agency, Robert C. Post, PhD, said that the findings that "have less support" require more research.

An unelected official at an agency supported by your tax dollars is saying that the most important research for reversing the obesity epidemic in this country is going to be ignored in favor of a "short and simple" message. What? Ignore the compelling studies that sugar is implicated in serious increases in death rates and instead offer a "simple" message to just eat less—instead of four doughnuts, only eat two? Does the government think Americans are too stupid to understand anything more complicated than that? How will we solve the obesity problem by simply eating less? If you're eating less and what

DR. ROCK REPORTS...
I'll Take My Vegetables in the Form of a Steak!

Vegetables are a good food in our diet, but don't be fooled that vegetables are the best food on your plate. They are far too low in essential amino acids and essential fatty acids to be the star players the "experts" say they are. All these vegetables are going to do is make you hungry and unsatisfied and push you toward starches and sweets—chips and cookies. And vegetables are still carbs! Instead of outing sugar, the government opted to heavily push vegetables.

Sometimes when I go to a restaurant, I won't order vegetables, just the steak. The waitress will often say, "No healthy vegetables, sir?"

Look! The cow ate tons more vegetable matter than I'll ever eat in a hundred lifetimes and turned it into the abundant essential macronutrients and micronutrients in the big juicy steak I'm about to enjoy. I guess you might say I'm the ultimate vegetarian.

---

you're eating is nutrient deficient, you will only be hungrier and eat more sugar!

The type of food matters, not just the amount. Not all calories are equal. For example, a calorie from an egg comes with the fat-soluble vitamins A, D, E, and K, the full spectrum of essential amino acids and B vitamins, and much more. This is anabolic food, making your muscles and bones stronger and you younger. A calorie from a carrot stick is practically devoid of amino acids and fat and is jokingly called *rabbit food*. Yes, there's beta-carotene, but we've previously shown all the populations that can't make use of this form of vitamin A. Now compare a calorie from a doughnut. The sugary doughnut triggers insulin for muscle teardown and fat storage. *And we're just scratching the surface here.* Look at the company this calorie keeps.

A bank robber is a man and so is a neurosurgeon, but these men are not equal in what they can contribute to society. To suggest that just "lowering calories" is the answer to epidemic muscle wasting and Sedentary Death Syndrome, Nutrient Deficiency Disorder, and obesity is an appalling and unconscionable slap in the face to nutritional science and the plight of the population. How about: "Just eat less rat poison"? It's just that irrelevant! Keeping it "simple" is good for industry profits, and what's more important than the politics of profit? Let's put *lobbying* in plain English. As an industry lobbies against peer-reviewed research, it is conducting business through bribery, kickbacks, and payoffs. Your health is under brutal attack in much the way the Mafia would do business—in this case, the Sugar Mafia.

Beware of sugar in all its many forms—as sweeteners for sodas, ketchup, barbecue sauce, ice creams, processed grains, and cereals. Even the slow-burning form from whole grains will spike insulin and trigger fat storage. For years, the sugar industry has hyped sugar as an energy source, but you can no longer look at a calorie as just another calorie in this era of Nutrient Deficiency Disorder. Every calorie you consume creates a metabolic consequence in your body. Five hundred calories of meat and eggs will cause anabolic fat burning and muscle toning; 500 calories of sugar and other high-glycemic carbs, like a white flour biscuit or a bowl of white rice, will create the metabolic consequence of fat storage and practically every disease you can name.

CHAPTER **21**

Glycation Nation
UNDERSTANDING WHY CARBOHYDRATES ARE
SUCH A "SWEET AND DANGEROUS" THREAT

Т he danger of sugar is not a new subject. As far back as the 1970s, in his book *Sweet and Dangerous*, John Yudkin, MD, former professor of nutrition at Queen Elizabeth College, London University, proved, in brilliant research worthy of the Nobel Prize, the truth about the risks of a diet high in carbohydrates. Dr. Yudkin demonstrated that the countries with the highest incidence of heart disease are the ones with the highest sugar intake (such as Britain and the United States), not those with the highest protein and fat consumption, as the late Ancel Keys, PhD, led people to believe. You'll recall Dr. Keys as the author of the disproven Seven Countries Study of 1958 mentioned in Chapter 17.

Dr. Yudkin's research was the first and some of the most conclusive to indicate that it was sugar, not saturated fat or cholesterol, that was causing the growing incidence of heart disease. He duplicated his findings repeatedly over a 30-year career.

It is unfortunate that Dr. Keys, while hyping his conclusions to journalists and politicians, repeatedly attacked Dr. Yudkin's findings. His ridicule of a fellow scientist was so successful that the many scientists who agreed with Dr. Yudkin and challenged the assumption that cholesterol was the cause of heart disease were labeled "Yudkin sugar quacks." These scientists were in the same position as Galileo when he proved, against the dogma of the Catholic Church and other scientists of the time, that Earth was *not* the center of the universe. The similarly dogmatic Cholesterol Cult muzzles those who don't agree with low-fat and high-carbohydrate cult dicta.

Glycation is a word Dr. Yudkin brought to our attention through his research with glycated hemoglobin in the 1970s. As one of the world's leading experts in carbohydrate metabolism, he showed that high levels of triglycerides, insulin, uric acid, cortisol, and blood pressure are all caused by high blood sugar.

Dr. Yudkin discovered that sucrose also weakened blood platelet cells, making them more prone to clotting. In this process called glycation, the sugar cross-links to protein structures such as red blood cells. In the simplest terms, high blood sugar coats your red blood cells, making them sticky and more prone to binding and attaching to artery walls.

When Dr. Yudkin first identified this phenomenon of glycation, he was 30 years ahead of his time. Today, these glycated protein and lipid molecules are called advanced glycation end products, or AGEs, an appropriate acronym because AGEs are what ages you. AGEs cause the age-related diseases of diabetes, heart disease, and dementia. These sticky AGEs interfere with intercellular signaling. They clog the arteries in your brain and cardiovascular system. They gum up the secretion and flow of your hormones. AGEs may cause cataracts, may trigger macular degeneration, and may even cause nerve damage leading to hearing loss and sensory integrity. AGEs are caused by high blood sugar, and they are linked to the *carbs and sugars* you eat!

When the sugar or carbohydrate nutrient is being digested in the stomach and small intestine, it breaks down into billions of dangerous single-oxygen atoms—missing a hydrogen electron—called free radicals. These unbalanced oxygen atoms course through your blood in nanoseconds, seeking to replenish the missing hydrogen atom they have lost. Right now, billions of these free radicals in your body are wreaking such havoc that, according to Dr. Bruce Ames, each cell in your DNA endures 10,000 free radical attacks a day. This produces more free radicals, as the injured cells are now unbalanced. This entire destructive process is called oxidative stress, an internal stress that you are so accustomed to feeling, you don't even realize you can prevent it. Nor do you realize that this oxidative stress is signaling the uncomfortable, early symptoms of aging and disease.

You can think of oxidative stress as the browning of your internal cellular structure, just as a sliced apple or peeled banana turns brown as it oxidizes in the open air. The visible cells are rapidly aging and dying. AGEs are this same phenomenon going on internally, and this glycation process interferes with the antiaging process of anabolism that we're offering to you. Everything from protein synthesis, to the repair of damaged organs and cells, to the protection of the eyes, organelles, and mitochondria is imperiled by AGEs.

SUGAR *AGES* YOU

The carbs and sugar that cause AGEs are recent food introductions to our species, and the political pressure on you to eat them is destroying the possibility of your good health. The greatest contributors to this dangerous level of runaway free radical damage and oxidative stress are refined sugar and grains. Do proteins and fats create AGEs? Not really.

According to microbiologist Sathya Schnell at the University of

Minnesota, "Of the three (proteins, fats, and carbohydrates), carbs are the biggest producer of free radicals. I won't say there aren't any fats or proteins that cause free radicals, but it would be like comparing a lake to the Pacific Ocean. I weighed a sugar cube and calculated how many nutrients were in it. It's roughly eight quadrillion—717 trillion and change. Then I multiplied that eight quadrillion by 11 for the approximate number of oxygen atoms in a single sugar cube. That would be approximately 88 quadrillion. Fats, on the other hand, are long carbon chains with just a couple of oxygen atoms on one end. Proteins are mostly amino acids with a few oxygen atoms. Therefore, fats and proteins are not significant sources of oxidative stress. Carbohydrates clearly are."

How many people are having just *one* sugar cube a day? Not many, because most people today consume about a quarter of a pound of sugar a day—75 pounds a year—and several tons in a lifetime. You don't use sugar? You use agave? You use honey or artificial sweeteners? Every form of sugar you know about causes the same harm as those packets of white sugar you put in your coffee.

Denham Harman, MD, PhD, of the University of Nebraska Medical Center, hypothesized the free radical theory of aging and disease in his laboratories a few years before Dr. Keys came up with his cholesterol-lipid hypothesis. Dr. Harman is in his nineties and still actively working to repeat his proof of this theory today. Many other scientists in biochemistry, microbiology, and molecular biology have also proved and are aligned with the free radical theory of aging and disease because of their own research, as well as the abundance of corroborative research in the field. This is not a hypothesis that is being *sold* to you, backed by for-profit industries. It's a theory that is in the process of being proved repeatedly in peer-reviewed scientific studies, in line with the scientific method.

"Over the past 7 years," says Ray D. Strand, MD, author of *What Your Doctor Doesn't Know about Nutritional Medicine May Be Killing You,* "I have reviewed well over 2,000 medical and scientific studies in regards to nutritional supplements and their effect on your health. These studies appearing in medical journals like the *New England Journal of Medicine, Journal of the American Medical Association, Lancet,* and *Annals of Internal Medicine* report that beyond any doubt the 'root' cause of well over 70 chronic degenerative diseases is 'oxidative stress.'"

Dr. Ames explains, "Mitochondrial decay with age due to oxidation of RNA/DNA, proteins, and lipids, is a major contributor to aging and the degenerative diseases of aging."

Timothy J. Smith, MD, author of *Renewal: The Anti-Aging Revolution,* says, "Dr. Harman's Free Radical Theory ranks with Galileo's invention of the telescope, Newton's discovery of gravity, and Einstein's theory of relativity. No breakthrough has had more profound implications for human health and longevity. . . . Dr. Harman deserves the Nobel Prize for his revolutionary work."

We could give you similar testimonies from 37 pages of doctors and scientists like these. Robert Lustig, MD, is another supporter of Dr. Yudkin's findings. Speaking about the late British nutritionist in a 2009 lecture titled "Sugar: The Bitter Truth," Dr. Lustig said, "Every single thing" that Dr. Yudkin warned about sugar in his 1972 book *Pure, White and Deadly* "has come to pass."

Dr. Lustig's lecture has gone viral and sparked coverage in the *New York Times* and on *60 Minutes.* In it Dr. Lustig argues that the USDA, American Heart Association, and American Medical Association based their recommendation of reduced dietary fat on the "immensely flawed science" behind Ancel Keys's Seven Countries Study.

Dr. Lustig says the low-fat craze that swept the country in the late 1980s and '90s led to the diabetes crisis today: "The problem is, when you remove the fat from processed food, it tastes like cardboard. In order to make it palatable, food companies added sugar, particularly HFCS [high-fructose corn syrup]. So we have had our food supply adulterated, contaminated, poisoned, tainted, on purpose, and we've allowed it . . . through the addition of fructose for palatability and ostensibly as a 'browning agent,' which has its own issues. Because, why it browns so well with the sugar in it is actually what's going on in your arteries [through glycation] . . . and contributing to atherosclerosis."

In studies, Dr. Lustig says, Dr. Yudkin proved that someone eating more than 110 grams of sugar per day was five times more likely to have a heart attack than someone eating less than 60 grams a day.

Did you catch that? If you consume more than 110 grams of sugar a day, as opposed to less than 60 grams a day, you are five times more likely to have a heart attack. But how many people are eating less than 110 grams of sugar a day?

This question is answered in the August 2009 issue of *Circulation,* a journal of the American Heart Association: For American women, the AHA recommends no more than 100 calories of sugar a day, which is 6 teaspoons, or 25 grams. For American men, it recommends no more than 150 calories a day, which is 9 teaspoons, or 38 grams.

One can of soda typically contains approximately 39 grams of sugar, which equals a full 9 teaspoons when extracted from the liquid. How many people are having a can of soda several times a day? The indulgence of a Starbucks Grande Caramel Frappuccino with whipped cream yields about 15 teaspoons of sugar, or 64 grams. An Arizona Energy drink contains 52 grams, which is just under the safe limit of 60 grams, so you might think you're doing something good for yourself with this choice, but you're not.

Consuming 110 grams or more in one day is frighteningly easy to do, and the average person could consume hundreds of grams of sugar a day.

This anti-nutrient appears in many guises, and according to Barnet Meltzer, MD, in his book *Food Swings,* it's wise to avoid them all: candies, chocolates, cake, ice cream, doughnuts, pastries, jams and jellies, and artificial sweeteners such as mannitol, saccharine, Equal, and NutraSweet, plus the refined white sugar present in brown sugar and turbinado sugar. And it's not just sucrose that's dangerous, but also refined grains, such as white rice, pasta, and processed cereals, because all of these act just like sugar and raise your blood sugar. In Italy, where pasta is queen, researchers are studying the dangers of refined grains. From their research, Denise Mann reported on CNN.com that "women who eat more white bread, white rice, pizza, and other carbohydrate-rich foods . . . are more than twice as likely to develop heart disease than women who eat less of those foods."

A THIEF BY ANY OTHER NAME

As high-fructose corn syrup loses its peachy position as the all-purpose cheap sweetener that industry brought to our government's open arms, the spin doctors of advertising are attempting to bring white sugar back, all dressed up like the bride and veiled as being healthy. Raise your antennae on all this hoopla over the removal of high-fructose corn syrup as many food manufacturers tout their virtue in replacing it with white or brown sugar, as if they were performing a service for your health.

White sugar is not a health food! And neither is molasses, blackstrap molasses, brown sugar, honey, or agave. All raise blood sugar levels and spike insulin the same way. Implying that any of these sugars is preferable is like implying that that there is a form of healthy cocaine. Sugar could be in the same category as cocaine and cigarettes. All refined carbohydrates, and especially the carbs in this quick-acting form, are the greatest killers. The most heinous crime has been to peddle all these sugars to us for over 100 years.

The fact is, fructose cannot be burned as glycogen in the muscle and is not a fuel for the brain, which burns only the glucose your liver produces. Fructose converts more quickly to fat than other sugars, which is why we've become a fatter nation on all this high-fructose corn syrup.

It's fat that turns off the appetite hormone ghrelin, not any form of sugar.

PART SIX

Foods That Keep You Young for Life

22

Eggs: The Gold Standard of Proteins

THERE IS SIMPLY NO MORE NUTRITIOUS, ACCESSIBLE, AND AFFORDABLE FOOD FOR THE ANABOLIC LIFE.

The highest biological value protein—the gold standard against which all other proteins are measured—is the whole egg. This is the best protein you can eat for anabolism because it contains the highest quantities of valine, leucine, and isoleucine, as well as *all* the other essential amino acids *in quantity.* Valine, leucine, and isoleucine— the branched-chain amino acids (BCAAs)—are essential to human life. They become particularly involved when you are under stress and at risk of breaking down lean muscle. They are used in energy and are metabolized primarily by muscle. When your body is under stress, whether from daily life, exercise, relationships, or more extreme circumstances, such as surgery, infections, burns, or fever, it will always require proportionately more BCAAs than other amino acids, and more leucine than either valine or isoleucine. One egg contains about 400 milligrams of leucine and 400 milligrams of valine and isoleucine. This is what scientists consider the ideal proportion for anabolism.

The egg is historically the perfect food, balanced with equal amounts of the highest quality amino acids and fats. This is another key you need to seek for anabolism: equal quantities of protein and fat in a whole food. If the fat is too low or the protein is too high, the food is out of balance and less digestible. This is why low-fat foods are simply *not* ideal for anabolism. When Americans ate the traditional American breakfast, up until the 1950s, which consisted of *whole* eggs, sometimes accompanied by bacon or sausage, we had far less obesity and practically no diabetes.

TWO EGGS A DAY CAN MAKE BELLY FAT GO AWAY

In the October 2008 issue of the *International Journal of Obesity,* scientists compared the weight-loss effect of eating an egg breakfast with a bagel breakfast. The study subjects, both overweight or obese men and women, ate either eggs or bagels for breakfast. Afterward, both groups ate roughly the same number of calories for the remainder of their daily meals. At the end of the study, the researchers found that the people who had eaten egg-based breakfasts had lost more fat and reported greater feelings of satiety than the people who had eaten bagels for breakfast. The researchers also found no difference in the cholesterol levels of the subjects, despite the fact that eggs are rich in cholesterol. This supports the now widely held theory that the cholesterol gained from eating a few eggs every day will have no negative impact on cholesterol levels.

Eggs are the only whole food that contain ample amounts of both vitamin A and vitamin D. Without the fat-soluble vitamins A, D, E, and K, you cannot assimilate other nutrients. All of these vitamins, taken from this one food—the egg—keep your skin young, which in itself is quite telling: When your skin looks good, that's a sign that the rest of your organs (those on the inside) are being repaired and rejuvenated properly.

Eggs may prevent breast cancer, too. A study reported by the American Association for Cancer Research found that women who consumed at least six eggs per week lowered their risk of breast cancer by 44 percent. You want the benefit of vitamin D from eggs, the very best source of natural vitamin D$_3$.

Eggs also contain selenium, which, like vitamin E, is an important part of the antioxidant process that protects cells from free radical oxidation. In many states in the country, and especially in the southern states, the soil is deficient in selenium. In 1997, an important study at Cornell University in Ithaca, New York, showed that an increase of selenium in the diet is a powerful measure for cancer prevention. In a 10-year study of groups of people who took a selenium supplement, as opposed to groups who took a placebo, rates of cancer were reduced by 41 percent in the selenium-supplemented groups. Recently, lawyer Jonathan Emord won a legal battle against the FDA to allow nutraceutical companies to include this information on the label of their selenium supplements:

"Selenium may reduce the risk of bladder, colon, prostate, and thyroid cancers. Scientific evidence concerning this claim is inconclusive. Based on its review, FDA does not agree that selenium may reduce the risk of these cancers."

Emord is the author of *The Rise of Tyranny* and *Global Censorship of Health Information,* and we consider him a modern-day hero.

Eggs are the most readily available food source for the important antioxidants for eye health: lutein and zeaxanthin. According to one

Marilyn's Message...

I believe the egg is a sexy food. It was the first protein I added back into my diet in quantity, and I actually felt the sexual benefits. I can honestly say that I went from somewhat frigid on plant protein to quite warm and cuddly on eggs. This is because eggs are one of the highest sources of choline, a nutrient suspected of enhancing the muscle contractions that increase sexual pleasure. The egg yolk delivers more choline than any other protein source. Choline is also available in beef (especially in the liver and kidney), pork, caviar, fish, and other seafood.

If you want to feel more sexually satisfied, I can tell you from my own experience that you need to eat more eggs. Eggs are a woman's best friend for other reasons, too: They are rich in vitamins A and K, and they contain zinc, which may also contribute to beautiful skin.

Eggs provide nutrients that regulate brain function, the nervous system, and the cardiovascular system; they bolster the immune system and help heal wounds. They are rich in B vitamins and minerals, including sulfur, which is essential for healthy hair and nails.

study, eating an egg a day may prevent age-related macular degeneration, a condition that destroys your sharp, central vision. Eggs are the ultimate convenience food. They are a quick meal solution, and they're affordable. They taste best if they're organic. Eggs from free-walking and cage-free hens are exceptional. These are more available than ever before, as egg farmers perfect their art. Eggs are excellent for breakfast, lunch, or dinner, *every day,* in myriad ways. One large egg contains 6 grams of high-quality protein, all the essential and nonessential amino acids, and less than 6 grams of fat. One large egg has fewer than 100 calories. Have as many as you want. You really can't overdo it on eggs.

CHAPTER 23

Dairy Power

MILK, CHEESE, AND YOGURT ARE MUSCLE
BUILDERS, BUT BEWARE: THESE FOODS ARE
HIGH IN CALORIES.

Dairy products follow eggs in this book for a reason: They fall second in the gold-standard measurements of high nutritional value foods, just a percentage point behind eggs. This discussion leaves out all the newfangled, messed-with, low-fat versions that were brought to us in the 1990s. None of those are *whole* foods. Nature made whole dairy for a reason. Otherwise, we'd have cows that naturally provided 2 percent or fat-free milk.

For your goal of fat loss, beware of the carbohydrates in milk. Milk is an anabolic food, but it carries with it a drawback for adults wishing to tone up and lose fat. When we did our research on both raw and pasteurized milk in our diet, we noticed significant fat gain, even from raw milk. If you're going to drink milk, watch your intake, and also cut your calories from other foods way back. In this program, since we focus on preserving and developing a toned body that shows attractive definition, we recommend that you be careful with milk, because if you're carbohydrate sensitive, which most of us are, you will stop fat burning and start sugar burning from the carbohydrates in milk. A glass of whole milk contains 12 grams of carbohydrates, 8 grams of protein, and 8 grams of fat.

WHOLE YOGURT AND KEFIR FROM COWS, SHEEP, OR GOATS

Yogurt, specifically, is an international staple in the healthy diet. Throughout the centuries, it has been one of the most important fermented foods and highly valued for longevity. The probiotics in yogurt can strengthen your immune system and bring you to a far higher level of health, especially when you include yogurt in your daily diet. Whole yogurt and kefir, rather than milk, are our preferred dairy choices. These are naturally occurring foods that self-create when whole, unlike raw milk, which begins to sour. The souring is caused by the formation of the *Lactobacillus* probiotics, the friendly bacteria you need for a clean stomach and digestive tract. Natural fermentation can't happen when milk is pasteurized to extend shelf life. Unfortunately, the friendly bacteria are destroyed by heat.

However, when pasteurized milk is used to make yogurt, the

probiotics form again. Commercial and organic yogurts and kefirs that contain the various probiotics will say so on their labels. With 30 percent of the daily calcium value in 1 cup, yogurt is considered a better source of calcium than a glass of pasteurized milk. Whole yogurt is digestible and is the healthiest alternative to pasteurized milk we have, and up to 2 cups a day is perfectly fine. Eat yogurt alone or with raw vegetables as a delicious afternoon snack, or in a salad at lunch, or even as an anabolic recharge right before you go to sleep. The friendly bacteria in yogurt help convert lactose to lactic acid in your intestines. This makes it easier to digest and less likely to cause the pain and discomfort of lactose intolerance.

A study led by Eileen Hilton, MD, in the *Annals of Internal Medicine* recommends just 1 cup of yogurt a day to add the *Lactobacillus acidophilus* to your digestive system. Another study, at the University of Tennessee, Knoxville, recommends 18 ounces to lose belly fat. In more complex terms, *L. acidophilus* ferments sugars. When this fermentation happens, yeast cannot use the sugar as the fuel that it needs to grow. When the sugar is fermented, it's made into lactic acid. Lactic acid lowers pH levels within the body, and when this happens, yeast cannot survive. Additionally, yogurt has been shown in several studies to provide increased vaginal health, specifically in the treatment of yeast infections. If you suffer from yeast infections, be sure to cut out sugar and processed (white) flour because yeast just loves to feed and propagate on sugar.

When home remedies actually work, they're always more beneficial for your health, as well as your wallet. It's always good to know exactly what you are putting into your body, and in the case of yogurt, it's something healthy. Georges Halpern, MD, PhD, an adjunct professor in the Department of Internal Medicine at the University of California, Davis, discovered that people who ate 2 cups of yogurt a day for 4 months increased the level of gamma interferon, which is a protein that helps your white blood cells fight off disease. Gamma interferon is one of the best defenses your body has against viruses, including the herpes virus. Studies have also shown that yogurt can help fight against bacterial infections, namely salmonella, and can be used when recovering from food poisoning. In all cases, we're suggesting unsweetened (or plain) whole-fat yogurt.

From infancy on, we're faced with many threats to the healthy balance of beneficial bacteria and infectious bacteria in our intestines.

During birth, a cesarean section deprives an infant of gathering its first supply of friendly bacteria from the mother while passing through the birth canal. The excessive use of antibiotic drug treatments destroys your probiotic balance. The word *antibiotic* means "anti-life." Antibiotics destroy probiotics, so after taking antibiotics it is critical to eat plenty of whole, unsweetened yogurt or drink unsweetened kefir to restore your probiotic population. It is important to understand that your beneficial bacteria play such a vital role in your overall health that you must supply them regularly.

Do you suffer from frequent stomachaches? You may be harboring *Helicobacter pylori* in your stomach—an ulcer-causing bacteria that is usually treated with large doses of antibiotics. However, there is evidence that eating lots of live-active-culture yogurt keeps ulcer-causing bacteria under control.

Are you plagued by constipation? This is a serious condition often caused by low-fiber, low-liquid diets. Constipation can lead to colon cancer. Yogurt's friendly bacteria take up residence in the gut and begin to compete with the harmful bacteria. You should choose yogurt as your go-to breakfast food rather than cereals and bread, which turn to sugar in your gut. Yogurt will foster a healthier environment in your intestines and lead to a longer and healthier life.

CHAPTER 24

Beef and Other Red Meats

POWERHOUSE PROTEINS FOR FUELING WEIGHT-LOSS AND MUSCLE GROWTH

At least weekly, a nutrition blogger writes another beef-bashing tirade—a journalistic drive-by shooting that causes another red meat scare among the readers who believe the writer's authority. These misled people then shun red meat for the poisonous choices of soy, sweets, cereals, all forms of dough, anemic chicken breasts, and lettuce. It's gotten to the point where if you are a meat eater, you often feel you have to lie about it or apologize. The nutritional vigilantism against beef in this country is one of the reasons we decided to write this book and set the record straight. Beef in all its forms is one of the most important foods you can eat for anabolism! We could not have restored our bodies without it.

Without beef and other red meats, you're at risk of damaging your chromosomes, because in all likelihood you have B_{12} and B_6 deficiencies. Beef packs a formidable nutrient wallop. This fact is at the foundation of this country's nutritional heritage. The legacy of leadership and innovation our forefathers left us was built on beef. People were attracted to our shores from all over the world because of our abundance of food and access to quality nutrition, much of it provided by beef, with its plentitude of macronutrients and micronutrients. Beef actually makes you look more vital and radiant. It builds, shapes, and tones muscle. It feeds your mitochondria and brain cells, and it keeps you in the game—and ahead of the pack. The same is true of lamb.

Consuming beef and other red meats contributes to fat loss and strength; it provides powerful antioxidants and naturally occurring B vitamins. Now let's be clear on what is and what is not red meat. Beef, bison, buffalo, venison, and lamb are easy to spot. Pork is also a red meat, as is all dark-meat poultry, including chicken, turkey, goose, and duck. What defines red meat is whether the muscle fibers contain the protein myoglobin. It's partially the myoglobin in these proteins that makes them anabolic winners. As you exercise, your muscles use up the oxygen that's stored in them. Myoglobin replenishes that oxygen. You're told to fill almost half your plate with antioxidant-rich vegetables. Grass-fed livestock graze on *tons* of plant food each month. Those vegetable nutrients are amazingly concentrated in the meat. When you pile vegetables on your plate, enjoy the colors, tastes, and textures, but look to get your nutrient advantage from meat and its fat. Two essential nutrients for human survival—saturated fat and high

Marilyn's Message...

Rock and I were confirmed vegetarians and then vegans, both for health and philosophical reasons, for more years than we care to count. Both of us recognized the degeneration of our bodies over time as a result of this way of eating. Newbie vegetarians are full of the thrill of the choice but not yet aware of the nutrient deficiencies, muscle wasting, and fat storage on their bodies. They will feel it as the years progress. We understand your programmed resistance to red meat and specifically beef, so we make this case fully to help you realize what you're giving up in health and appearance if you resist including protein in your anabolic diet.

biological value protein—are nonexistent in vegetables. Name a vegetable that provides sufficient levels of the branched-chain amino acids. You can't.

Beef and other red meats are loaded with vitamins and minerals. They are rich in phosphorus, which is important for strong teeth and bones; magnesium and potassium, which are vital for your heart; and thiamin, riboflavin, niacin, and vitamin B_{12}.

The very last thing you *ever* want to do is eat sugar on top of red meat. Eat enough meat so you're satiated and not craving dessert. Dessert is more an issue of eating too little fat than of craving sugar. You don't receive enough fat for satiety on a low-fat diet.

BEEF PREVENTS ANEMIA

Beef and other red meats are great providers of iron, which is an essential mineral because it is involved in every process of oxygen transport and all metabolic and protein synthesis processes in your body. There are two forms of iron available from your diet: heme and nonheme.

Heme iron is found only in red meats, poultry, and fish. The richest source of heme iron is liver. Nonheme iron is found in plants. The reason it is important to know this is because nonheme iron is not absorbed as well as heme iron. An iron deficiency will cause anemia. You need only to eat some beef or lamb regularly to provide enough iron to prevent anemia. If you're always tired, you should have your iron levels tested frequently because the symptoms of anemia are serious and it frequently goes undiagnosed.

Beef and other red meats provide vitamin B_{12} in greater abundance than even eggs. You won't find B_{12} anywhere in the vegetables on your plate. Vegetarians may attempt to argue this point, but it's inarguable. If they tell you to just leave the dirt on your vegetables for B_{12} or to eat sea vegetables, they're talking about analogues of B_{12} that are inferior and nonactive forms of the vitamin. Think about the idea of eating dirt for a nutrient advantage.

If you have a B_{12} deficiency, you can't absorb iron, so you risk getting anemia. Anemia on its own causes many symptoms, including fatigue, depression, psychosis, seizures, and loss of appetite. But anemia, with all of its many symptoms, is only the *first* on the long list of problems caused by a B_{12} deficiency, which together can lead to serious disorders and nerve damage.

A vitamin B_{12} deficiency is so harmful to your body that you simply can't risk the repercussions. It occurs most often in the elderly; in those who lack the intrinsic factor, a protein secreted in the stomach that allows for the absorption of vitamin B_{12}; and in those who refuse to eat any animal products. Vegans suffer from this disorder, and their symptoms are often visible, as they are unknowingly living in a state of vitamin B_{12} pernicious anemia. Pernicious anemia is the inability of your intestines to absorb B_{12}, whereas in iron deficiency anemia, your blood doesn't contain enough red blood cells. Supplementation with shots or pills is the treatment, but blood levels of vitamin B_{12} should be checked regularly to ensure the supplementation is adequate. The best method, however, is to include the natural sources of B_{12} in your diet.

Some symptoms of vitamin B_{12} deficiency include tingling and numbness in your hands and feet (caused by nerve damage), loss of balance, fatigue, pale skin, diarrhea, jaundice, swollen and sore or tingling tongue, light-headedness, and concentration problems. The B_{12} deficiency is a perfect example of the nutrient deficiencies of today becoming the diseases of tomorrow. Vegans and vegetarians, for the sake of your children, we implore you to take note.

ZINC OR EXTINCT

The mineral zinc is rarely, if ever, discussed openly in relation to sexuality and survival. There is no body repair without zinc. Have you had cosmetic surgery or any other surgery? Were you prescribed zinc for healing?

Leading molecular biologists today are concerned that at least 12 percent of Americans suffer from zinc deficiency, but government estimates have shown that up to 45 percent of adults over 60 are deficient in zinc. When zinc is deficient in human cells, there is considerable free radical damage to DNA, affecting health, reproduction, and longevity. A zinc deficiency negatively affects libido and sexual response. Zinc is also involved in healthy brain and reproductive development in children.

Because zinc is most plentiful in highly anabolic proteins such as oysters and beef and other red meats, it makes sense for you to eat these foods to ensure that you have plenty of this mineral.

I Can Get Zinc from Beans, Right?

Wrong. More likely, you'll have gas. According to research by Janet R. Hunt, PhD, RD, published in the *American Journal of Clinical Nutrition,* the bioavailability of zinc from vegetarian diets is lower than from non-vegetarian diets. The position of the American Dietetic Association and Dietitians of Canada on vegetarian diets, as published in the *Journal of the Academy of Nutrition and Dietetics,* is that since vegetarians typically eat high levels of soy, legumes, and whole grains, which contain phytates that bind zinc and inhibit its absorption, they will have a greater risk of zinc deficiency than meat eaters will. As we pointed out in Chapter 14, if you're eating grains, legumes, or beans with your zinc-rich proteins, the zinc will not be absorbed as well, if at all. Vegetables are a better side dish to go with meat.

Raise your zinc status with red meat to avoid zinc deficiency. It's a cosmetic mineral you simply can't live without. In less scientific terms, a zinc deficiency may cause stretch marks; small breasts; scoliosis; hypermobility in the joints, such as temporomandibular joint (TMJ); aged and loose skin because of reduced collagen; slow healing of wounds; and frequent infections. Maladies of the eyes, such as glaucoma, cataracts, nearsightedness, macular degeneration, and retinal detachment are all related to zinc deficiency.

Children and teenagers need zinc for normal development. Zinc deficiencies cause low body weight, poor appetite, rough skin, mental lethargy, short stature, and retarded puberty. Consuming beef will mean consuming the most readily accessible food with the highest amount of bioavailable zinc. So when you see steak, pot roast, brisket, short ribs, meat loaf, or any lamb dish, realize that you have the option for a zinc-rich meal. The chart on page 197 from the Linus Pauling Institute's Micronutrient Information Center at Oregon State University gives you a sense of the zinc content of popular proteins. Oysters are the highest on the list. Many of our oysters come from farmed oyster beds in Korea, and as of May 1, 2012, the FDA warned against the importation, sale, and consumption of Korean oysters, citing contamination with norovirus (from human feces), so we've lost a significant source of food high in zinc for the time being.

"Meat is the single richest source of iron and zinc and contributes significant amounts of vitamins," says Mary Abbott Hess, RD, MS, former president of the American Dietetic Association, in a *Time* magazine article from June 2001.

In steak and in olive oil, you receive stearic acid the way nature intended. The problem with olives, however, is that they're inedible unless they're cured. Cured means brine, and brine means salt, and salt causes water retention that gives you the doughboy look. So go for your stearic acid in steak and other red meat for the benefits you think you're getting from olives, but without all that salt.

PREVENT BRAIN DECAY WITH ALA

The recently rediscovered nutrient from red meat known as alpha lipoic acid (ALA) performs functions in your body much like an antioxidant and is both fat and water soluble. It was just 40 years ago that ALA was found not only to help convert blood sugar into energy, but also to act as an antioxidant. Unlike other antioxidants that are either fat soluble or water soluble, but not both, ALA is able to permeate all cell parts to neutralize free radicals. Neutralizing free radicals is crucial because free radical attacks on your cells age you more than any other process, according to the free radical theory of aging. And since your brain is made of phospholipids—fat and cholesterol—which are easily damaged by oxidation, free radical damage can happen quite easily. You don't want your brain under attack by anything, and this is the last area where you want to allow free radical damage.

ALA stands alone as an antioxidant in potency and absorbability precisely because of its water and fat solubility. The fat solubility is a unique attribute that allows it to protect your brain, specifically in preventing lipofuscin and peroxidation—which in simple terms is a process where age spots are caused by free radical damage in the brain. This is brain decay, and you can prevent it with ALA.

Researchers writing in the Nutrition Reporter newsletter called ALA quite possibly the "universal antioxidant." ALA equally protects your liver and other organs that require *water-soluble* antioxidants to combat oxidation. ALA also mimics insulin and therefore helps to control blood sugar. For people with type 2 diabetes, it may enhance the body's receptivity to insulin. ALA is also helpful for cardiovascular and mental health, liver function, general eye health, and maintaining a healthy immune system. It improves the body's ability to build lean body mass and reduce fat, and is therefore extremely valuable in overcoming obesity and preventing sarcopenia. Over the past few years, the pace of research into ALA has increased dramatically.

The nutrient advantage is about prevention. It's about giving yourself what you need to keep your body working like a finely tuned machine instead of breaking down. The discovery of this amazing antioxidant in beef is a discovery about prevention that you don't hear about in newspapers because they are filled with beef-bashing articles. Medical reporting has most often been tucked comfortably into bed with pharmaceuticals, but this can change through information. There is already an outcry from the ailing population for change. We hear it. You want to know *what works!*

GLUTATHIONE: KING OF THE ANTIOXIDANTS

What is glutathione? It's the body's most powerful natural antioxidant. Anything that increases its production is more valuable than money in the bank. And this is another major function of ALA: It *increases the production of glutathione.*

Highest Zinc Content in Proteins

FOOD	SERVING	ZINC
Oysters	6 medium (cooked)	76.3 mg
Beef	3 ounces (cooked)	6.0 mg
Dungeness crab	3 ounces (cooked)	4.7 mg
Turkey (dark meat)	3 ounces (cooked)	3.8 mg
Pork	3 ounces (cooked)	2.2 mg
Chicken (dark meat)	3 ounces (cooked)	1.8 mg

Glutathione occurs naturally in your body but diminishes as you age. One of its important functions is the detoxification of poisons in your liver. Since your liver is the chemical processing center, neutralizing, breaking down, directing, and eliminating every single chemical that passes through your body, it stands to reason that if your liver is healthy, there is a greater chance that your other organs will also be healthy.

Keeping your liver healthy keeps your heart and brain healthy. It's tragic that the statins prescribed to lower cholesterol can damage your liver. The medical focus on heart health overlooks this physiological truth. If you take many drugs, medicine can be the cause of more liver-taxing chemicals going into your body than anything else you do. For this reason, side effect warnings on drugs frequently advise against taking a drug if you suffer from liver disease. But in our society, with so many chemical pollutants in our food, air, and water, and with so many drugs in the medicine cabinet, you may actually be suffering from a liver disorder and not even realize it.

One thing is for sure: Pharmaceutical drugs overwork and overtax the liver. In addition to protecting your liver, the natural antioxidant glutathione protects your brain from free radical damage. An ALA deficiency may be associated with brain disorders such as stroke, dementia, Parkinson's, and Alzheimer's, so beef up! You want this nutrient in your bloodstream today to protect yourself from the diseases of tomorrow.

For many years, European physicians have been successfully treating type 2 diabetes with 600 to 1,200 milligrams of supplemental ALA

Marilyn's Message...

Most medical doctors know nothing about alpha lipoic acid (ALA) and how it can help preserve brain health and treat diabetes. The information comes from one of my father's postdoctoral students, Bruce Ames, PhD, of the University of California, Berkeley, a highly respected researcher who is still hard at work in his eighties. Dr. Ames is looking at your health on the molecular level through the eyes of a professor of biochemistry and molecular biology. Physicians, by contrast, are trained to hunt for disease and fight symptoms with drugs. The difference is enormous! One is observing the positive effect of nontoxic nutritional solutions that protect the body and create optimal functioning on the molecular level, which means *health.* The other is trained in disease identification and treatment. The medical doctor is trained to do battle on the terrain called your body in the "war on cancer," with heroic measures such as surgery and the use of radiation and chemotherapy—the slash-and-burn approach. He is trained to address the biggest killer we have—heart disease—with radical bypasses, now shown to be a failing procedure, rather than with nutrient enhancements.

Rock and I owe a debt of gratitude to Dr. Ames for the discoveries of ALA and the neuroprotective antioxidant acetyl-L-carnitine, which we knew nothing about until his work came into the journals. Rock and I share the opinion that Dr. Ames is one of the greatest molecular biologists of our time. He leaves his labs to take constant interviews to warn the public in simple language that our nutrient deficiencies of today are our diseases of tomorrow.

You need ALA and acetyl-L-carnitine, and this need is met in your diet best when there is adequate animal protein. As a vegetarian who gave up all red meats and other animal proteins for over 20 years, I now eat red meat plentifully, and I know firsthand the youthful repair this brings to my body. I can see it and I can feel it. If you're not a meat eater, or even if you are a meat eater and want the benefit of this remarkable brain-sustaining nutrient combination, you can take it in supplement form. Dr. Ames himself takes a daily dose of 400 milligrams of ALA and 1,000 milligrams of acetyl-L-carnitine to prevent brain decay. So do we!

per day. If you have diabetes or prediabetes (also known as metabolic syndrome), you may wish to share this successful medical treatment with your physician to see whether it's right for you.

If you wish to prevent diabetes and other serious nutrient deficiencies, as well as to lose the fat that is covering your toned muscles, you'll want to eat red meat only with vegetables—not with starches of any kind, not even sugar in your coffee or an artificial sweetener in anything at that meal.

IF YOU'VE BEEN TOLD IT'S BAD, IT'S PROBABLY GOOD FOR YOU

It takes an open mind to realize that so much of what you've been told about nutrition and your health may be wrong, and we've only just begun. At the beginning of this program, we promised to make you an expert on why your diet must include such condemned foods as butter, eggs, and plenty of red meat. But we still must counteract the programming that brought you to be fearful of these foods. Meanwhile, now that we've covered the most anabolic and cosmetic macronutrients—the saturated fats and whole proteins—the proof will come to you in the *doing*. Only *you* can convince yourself of how the anabolic foods will complement your exercise efforts and bring the many benefits your body requires to end obesity and sarcopenia.

PART SEVEN

Making Our System Work in Your Life

CHAPTER 25

A New Way of Eating
RELEARN HOW TO FUEL WITH THE BASIC
GUIDELINES OF THE YOUNG FOR LIFE DIET.

W e are now in a food revolution, and we are writing to help propel forward the understanding that Nutrient Deficiency Disorder is a critical condition. As you travel around our country, you can see how unwell most of our people appear to be. Excess weight, soft and slumped bodies, obvious lack of energy, and prematurely aged faces are the norm. As you follow the Young for Life program and apply the information we have shared, you will notice even more as you spring back to youthful vitality that together we must see this revolution through. There was no overwhelming concern about our fruit and vegetable intake in medicine, in government dietary guidelines, or in the American kitchen prior to 1985 and the publication of *Fit for Life*. There were only the first rumblings of the need for organic produce of any kind. As a population, we certainly didn't worry about the pesticides on our fruits and vegetables, or even know about something called "genetically modified food." The vegetables on our dinner plates were of the "convenience" variety—mostly frozen or canned.

Just as we paid little attention to vegetables before *Fit for Life,* the fuss over fruit was also minimal. Fruit was not shipped in great quantities all over the country, nor was it imported. We had what grew in our regions, and regional choices were basically what we saw in our supermarkets. We all ate plenty of watermelon on the Fourth of July, to launch the greater consumption of summer fruits. But often, rather than eating fresh fruit, we ate fruit salads canned in sugary syrup. We squeezed oranges by hand to make fresh orange juice. In fact, it is likely that the majority of people favored cooked or canned fruit over fresh. Fresh peaches, plums, blueberries, and cherries ended up in cobblers and pies, and strawberries became homemade jam or the topping on strawberry shortcake.

I was fortunate because I grew up with a different experience. I lived in France as a young teenager, and I learned firsthand of the love of fresh salads and a wide array of techniques to produce amazing vegetable dishes. From 1975 to 1998, I brought my love for innovative vegetable dishes to the vegetarian, vegan, and raw food movements. However, I have never enjoyed my daily meals in my entire life as much as I enjoy the diet that makes me young for life. I'm excited to share it with you! I want you to experience firsthand the reality that there are foods that age and tire or depress you, and foods that energize and rejuvenate you. In this and the next two chapters, you'll find my own personal way of eating, which I have developed by trial and error, honed, and brought to this level. This approach keeps me feeling strong and wonderful. You'll have your variations, and I encourage you to develop your own style. I'm offering my personal template to launch you into what I have found to be the most beneficial, practical, and palate-pleasing direction.

BASIC GUIDELINES

1. Avoid dehydration.

According to the Mayo Clinic, depending on your body composition, you are about 60 percent water. Your brain and muscles are 75 percent water; your bones are 22 percent water.

If you're not adequately hydrated, you're risking joint pain, a toxic body, high blood pressure, asthma, constipation, dry and wrinkled skin, sunken eyes, dark circles under your eyes, brittle hair and nails, and so much more. The Mayo Clinic notes that your body requires water as its "principle chemical component" for every one of your body systems.

Your blood contains 5 quarts of water. You must replenish this water every day. Not all 5 quarts! But if you're not drinking enough water for your body's needs, your blood will not be hydrated sufficiently, and you're going to pay the price. Adequate water intake ensures that sufficient nutrients will be transported to your cells. Adequate water keeps your lymph system working expeditiously to collect cellular waste. Hyaluronic acid in your skin absorbs the water you drink to keep your skin cells plump and your skin free from the lines and grooves that signal premature aging. (Just that one highly visible symptom may be enough to convince you to drink plenty of water.) But fat loss is dependent on adequate water intake as well. If you're dehydrated, your body will be overly acidic and you'll store, rather than flush, the fat.

"Eight glasses a day" is the traditional recommendation, but you may find that you need more. Since caffeine in tea, coffee, and chocolate and vegetables like asparagus are diuretics, when these come into your diet, drink more water. In addition to water, you can drink other hydrating fluids, including coconut water, naturally bubbly mineral waters, and iced or hot herbal teas. Whether the weather is cold or hot, fluid intake should be your primary focus. After air, water is the second most important nutrient.

If you're off the mark right now on at least eight glasses of water per day, you can get there. Here's how.

• First thing in the morning, slowly drink 16 ounces of water or two cups of noncaffeinated herbal tea. This may sound like a lot, but it's one of the best ways to "get things moving quickly" before you head out the door. The weight of the water spurs the colon to action.

• Before a meal, try to drink a glass of water. Your digestive juices are liquid and if you're dehydrated, your body will "borrow" from organs, such as your lungs or heart, to make digestive juices; thus, the known fact that dehydration causes asthma and high blood pressure. An additional perk to preventing these common problems is that you'll eat less food if you stay sufficiently hydrated.

• Whenever you take supplements, drink water. Many need to be taken with food, though, so take the supplement when you drink your glass of water directly before your meal.

• Begin to cut your water intake by dinner, or you'll be up during the night urinating.

• Keep water close to you at night and don't allow yourself to be thirsty. Take a few sips of water.

• If you are hungry between meals, first drink a glass of water or herbal tea because dehydration can mask itself as hunger. If after having water or herbal tea, you're still hungry, honor your body's call for nutrients and eat an anabolic snack.

2. Eat regularly.

Going without food is another problem. You'll go straight into Nutrient Deficiency Disorder (NDD), fat storage, and muscle wasting when you do. Your body is made of molecules that it needs for all the processes it handles. It is constantly removing worn-out cells made of molecules, and it constantly requires the raw material to build new ones. You're the foreman of your body and you must provide those molecules by feeding your cells. Otherwise, you're forcing your body to tear down muscle.

If you want to lighten up for a day or two, eat more raw and cooked vegetables, blended salads, nuts, yogurt, and fish. A lack of food won't rest the body. You rest the body with meditation and sleep. A few days of lighter eating, if you choose, can still maintain adequate nutrients in your body. But notice that you'll be hungrier, you may crave sugar, and your body may also quickly seem less toned. Lightening up is a short-term option. We eat regularly, but we eat small amounts as a rule, so we don't feel the need to lighten up.

3. Detoxify with C-Youth

Vitamin C detoxification is probably the most powerful form of detoxification. Vitamin C removes pollutants, protects against the free radical damage of radioactive poisons, and removes heavy metals, pathogenic bacteria, and viruses. This is the most biologically active and friendly way to detoxify based on your body's biochemical needs.

Our choice is C-Youth, a formula that contains the important mineral cofactors. We began with ¼ teaspoon (1,000 milligrams) in 1 ounce of water after each meal and before bed. We slowly worked up to 4,000 milligrams or more over 3 months, especially in flu season or when under stress. (The DRI is 2,000 milligrams per day, but higher doses can be therapeutic.) Experiment and see what works for you, but go slowly like we did to find your most comfortable level. C-Youth is available on marilyndiamond.com. This formula dates back nearly 50 years to the researchers who discovered this vitamin and understood the serious repercussions of vitamin C deficiency.

4. Stay off the scale.

This is not a weight loss program. It's a muscle-shaping, fat loss plan that will reward you with looking and feeling more youthful. We're not recommending that you strive for the gaunt look, which is a sign of premature aging, and no one wants you to suffer from obesity. We're offering you a way of eating the foods you need to keep shapely muscle and allow your body to overcome NDD and achieve your healthy normal weight.

We're helping you build into your body the *vitality* for moderate exercise. Our goal is that you have the energy and strength to be *more youthfully active*. As you know, lack of activity is a big risk factor for disease.

Forget the focus on weight loss. You're going to chart your success by looking in the mirror. You'll see your progress as your clothes first fit you better and then become looser.

Soon you'll be in clothes you once couldn't fit into, so don't throw out what you've reluctantly relegated to the back of the closet. You'll be back in your favorite dress or jeans sooner than you realize.

If you're already skinny, you'll see more muscle tone on your body. Just a 7 percent increase in your protein intake improves muscle tone, even if you're not working out.

5. Make it fun and satisfying.

This lifestyle begins with a 90-day carb-addiction-breaking system to turn you into a fat burner. Every 72 hours, you can have a "carb break" meal that includes starchy vegetables such as potatoes with the skin, whole yams, or winter squashes. Or if you're craving grain, this is a perfect time for your favorite brunch of pancakes or French toast, or your favorite sandwich on high-quality, high-fiber whole grain bread, or pasta, or rice— you'll know what you're craving. If you want a dessert, a good alternative is to have a sweet with tea in the afternoon like the Brits—all on its own— so you're not forming advanced glycation end products (AGEs) by putting sweets on top of protein at dinner. It's best to avoid desserts *because they're sugar,* but if you do indulge, take C-Youth or vitamin C afterward.

In all likelihood, on the Young for Life program you will not stop fat burning from one meal of carbs, and if you do, it will not be for long, as you're going right back to protein meals. You don't have to take the carb breaks if you're not craving them, but if you feel like you need one every 72 hours to stay on the program, we encourage you to take it. If you decide, like we did, to stop all carbs for 3 months, you'll probably see muscle tone faster, and you'll lose more fat and feel remarkably healthy and energetic, with an amazing renewal in your skin (and other cells). At the end of 3 months, your carb addiction will be broken. In our experience, carbs will have lost their power over you, and you will be completely in charge of when to have them.

Marilyn's Message...

What am I doing telling you to eat potatoes? We all know that they are a high-glycemic carb, and most experts ban them from the diet.

Eat the old-fashioned potato! Eat the skin, especially since it's loaded with vitamins, minerals, and fiber! It's the fiber that's necessary to lower the glycemic index (for great information on the GI, visit glycemicindex.com). With the peel, potatoes are a delicious and ancient whole food that pervades practically every culture. Their bad rap simply isn't justified.

Eat whole grains, like brown rice, if you prefer, but they're much newer in the human diet and require far more processing before they're edible. Plus, they contain a bran fiber that can be harsher than the fiber of the natural potato to the delicate strands of the villi in your small intestine, which serve to absorb the nutrients your body needs. It's a good idea to limit whole grains and to eat them infrequently. Remember, like any other carb, they break down into sugar, just more slowly. Skip them as much as possible.

THE LAW OF ATTRACTING GOOD QUALITY

The sky is falling! The sky is falling! Everything out there is bad for you! There's nothing left to eat!

Yes, there is! There is plenty to eat. We have amazing, wholesome food abundance in this country, and the more we deny this and bellyache over all that is wrong with our food and our environment, the worse it is for us. When you're stuck in this mode, you're in mental catabolism. We're speaking from experience. We've been through many phases when our philosophies made us quite inflexible about a wide variety of foods that didn't fit on our list.

On this program, we encourage you to turn a corner. Eat the anabolic foods, keep your focus on the anabolic exercises, take your supplements, and help put an end to Nutrient Deficiency Disorder, Sedentary Death Syndrome, and sarcopenia. Like us, you will see that a symptom of NDD is holding on to the depressing notion that there is nothing left that is good for you to eat.

The fact is, we're in an exciting era of tremendous change and progress! People are awake to the issues that must be changed, and knowledge is power. New solutions come when the largest numbers of people demand them. For example, 87 percent of Americans want genetically modified food labeled, so it *will* eventually be labeled—sooner rather than later if you speak out. Have this positive attitude and sign every petition.

Meanwhile, we have a greater abundance of fresh, local, and organic food than ever before. Heritage farming is a promising movement. The original varieties of many vegetables, such as tomatoes and greens, are now widely available. And farmers are also beginning to raise the original varieties of animals that were once on our menus. When you shop in the market or online, look for these options. Try to go to more than one market or to a local purveyor once in a while. You'll find high-quality produce and meat if you're looking for it. Many great deals on unusual items—iodine-rich sea vegetables and seaweeds; Asian mushrooms, greens, and cucumbers; and Asian and Indian herbs and spices—can be found at locally owned Asian or Indian family markets. We often shop in these markets, and in local Italian markets as well. We find lovely ingredients that make life in the kitchen so much more interesting.

If you're looking for quality, cleanliness, and ethically produced eggs and dairy, make your best effort to buy organic or heritage eggs from cage-free hens, and dairy from organic or family-owned companies that have been in business for a long time.

Many aged imported cheeses, such as Parmesan and varieties of Swiss cheese, are made from unpasteurized milk. Organic Valley produces raw cheeses that we find more digestible since they contain their natural enzymes. Wherever we're shopping, we buy what looks good to us at that time and fits into the plans for the food we're making on that day or in the days that follow. You never know when something new and interesting will catch your eye. Variety is the spice of life.

We enjoy dining in restaurants where food is often not organic. We especially love seafood restaurants because their fish is almost always fresher, and many we frequent offer wild-caught fish, our preference, and they prepare fish with techniques that are hard to duplicate in the home kitchen. It cuts into the easy flow of our very enjoyable lives to be manic on such details as whether a food is organic.

THE NUTRIENT ADVANTAGE GUIDE

E Carbs: **potatoes in skins,** high-fiber grains (especially rye or raw oat muesli), legumes; only if desired and only every 72 hours

D Low-sugar fruits: **green apples,** grapefruits, **blueberries, strawberries, blackberries;** all fruits in moderation—once a day or less

C **White meat poultry,** low-fat fish cooked in butter, **raw almonds, flaxseeds,** hazelnuts, Brazil nuts, walnuts, pecans, macadamias, cashews, **peanuts, almond and other nut butters,** sugar-free chocolate and carob

B Vegetables: avocados, **tomatoes, cucumbers, bell peppers,** onions, leeks, shallots, garlic, **spinach,** carrots, celery, baby lettuces, romaine lettuce, all leafy greens, green and yellow string beans, summer squash, eggplant, artichokes, cabbage, cauliflower, broccoli, winter squash, fresh and dried herbs (thyme, oregano, parsley, sage, marjoram, bay leaf, basil, rosemary, dill), and spices (chiles, curries, turmeric, cayenne, cinnamon, nutmeg, cardamom, allspice, etc.)

A **Whole eggs, butter, red meat** (including beef, lamb, dark meat poultry, natural pork), heavy cream, crème fraîche, sour cream, **raw cheese,** mozzarella cheese, low-salt cheeses, imported cheeses, **whole plain yogurt,** nitrite-free cured meats (such as sausages, bacon, salami, pâté, liverwurst, and ham), all fatty fish and seafood (such as **salmon, tuna,** mackerel, sea bass, oysters, shrimp, crab, lobster, smoked salmon and herring, caviar, and all fish roe), extra-virgin olive oil, **unfiltered olive oil,** and virgin coconut oil

NOTE: Eat more "A" foods and less of the other categories as you move up the pyramid toward "E." Buy free-range, grass-fed, or organic versions of those items in bold if possible. Fish should be wild caught, if available.

Marilyn's Message...

"Eat your vegetables!" Of course you would expect to hear this from the author of *Fit for Life*. But there are three caveats for receiving the benefits of vegetables.

• They do not have to be raw; sometimes it is far better to cook them.

• Don't eat too many with meat. Vegetables bring a lot of water into the stomach. If you eat too many at your meal with an anabolic protein, the extra water from the vegetables may impede digestion and make you feel bloated.

• Eat a reasonable serving. The suggestion that you must have more vegetables on your plate than any other food is not an anabolic choice. No need to go crazy. You're not a rabbit.

Carrots actually yield more nutrients after they've been cooked, since their nutrients are bound up in the fiber or cellulose that the human digestive tract does not break down. Beware of eating too many coarse, raw, high-fiber vegetables with your anabolic protein choices. You'll sweep out your nutrient advantage.

Also, salads are not mandatory every day or at every meal. There are plenty of easy recipes in this program for fabulous vegetable dishes. It's a matter of preference. The point I'm making is that warm veggies and cold are seasonal choices. Summer demands many more salads. Winter appreciates warm food.

In our relaxed approach to our food, we do very well—far better than when we're fanatical! Just stay with your anabolic foods, your exercises, and your supplements. And have a good time!

Our meal recommendations allow for you to eat plenty of vegetables—probably far more than you've been eating. The good news is these guidelines allow you to maintain recommended levels of no more than 60 grams of carbohydrates a day, as established by the late John Yudkin, MD, professor of nutrition at Queen Elizabeth College, London University. At this level, you remain in fat-burning mode and out of the zone for increased risk for heart disease.

CARBS IN VEGETABLES

VEGETABLE	Carbs (grams)	VEGETABLE	Carbs (grams)
Artichoke (whole globe)	10.3	Onions	7.9
Artichoke hearts	2.0	Peas	9.3
Asparagus	4.11	Potato (boiled with skin)	20.13
Broccoli	7.18	Potato (baked with skin)	21.55
Brussels sprouts	7.10	Potato skin (medium, plain)	10.0
Butter lettuce	1.2	Pumpkin	4.9
Cabbage, green	5.5	Radish	3.43
Cabbage, red	3.7	Romaine lettuce	1.7
Carrots	8.22	Spinach	3.75
Carrots (raw)	9.58	Squash, butternut	10.49
Cauliflower	4.11	Squash, spaghetti	6.46
Celery (5" stalk)	0.5	Sweet potato (baked)	20.71
Chard, Swiss	4.13	Tomatoes	3.89
Cucumber (unpeeled)	3.63	Tomatoes (canned)	4.0
Eggplant	8.73	Tomatoes (cherry)	2.2
Kale	5.63	Yam (baked)	26.99
Mushrooms	3.26	Zucchini	2.69
Okra	3.0		

The chart above shows the carbohydrate count for fresh vegetables. You'll see that you can eat plenty and not reach 60 carbs a day. Fiber in fresh vegetables reduces the impact of the carbs on your blood sugar. Carb counts are for cooked or raw vegetables, since not all are eaten raw. Each count is for ⅔ cup or less of vegetables.

One small baked potato in the skin will have around 21 grams of carbs. If you wish to lower the carbs, scoop out some of the potato and season the skin with garlic butter and salt. Drizzle boiled fingerlings or new potatoes with a little olive oil and salt. Or toss some steamed red potatoes in butter and salt and enjoy them with your eggs. Think of carbs in approximately ½-cup servings to make sure the carb portion on your plate is about half of the protein you're eating.

FRUIT

Fruit sugar is fructose, which is most easily stored as fat. The likelihood that you've already eaten enough carbs to have plenty for muscle fuel means excess fruit will be converted to triglycerides and stored as fat. The important word here is *excess*. When we ate mostly fruit in our raw food diets, although we were skinny, we were also fat.

In this program, it's best to limit your intake to one serving a day of low-sugar fruit, such as a bright green apple or deep-colored berries. There may be days when you eat more, especially in the summer. During those times, become more active quickly; otherwise, you're going to be wearing that fruit as pudginess. If you have diabetes, you may wish not to eat any fruit at all until you've dropped your blood sugar and sought your doctor's assistance to lower your insulin. At the end of 90 days, you'll have regulated your fruit consumption by eating it in moderation. Fruit, after all, is a sugar, and in this era of obesity and diabetes, we must reduce all sugars to prevent the explosive and costly rise in these epidemics.

Here are the carb counts for certain fresh fruits.

CARBS IN FRESH FRUIT

FRUIT	Carbs (grams)	FRUIT	Carbs (grams)
Avocado (½)	8.5	Cantaloupe (½ cup)	6.36
Banana (small)	23.07	Cherries (½ cup)	11.05
Blackberries (½ cup)	6.82	Green apple (1)	14.0
Blueberries (½ cup)	10.73	Watermelon (½ cup)	5.74

DRINK YOUR ANTIOXIDANTS

You can feel quite flawless in the morning just by starting your day, no matter how early, with antioxidant-rich tea, because you are saturating your body first thing with powerful, free radical fighters. There are many blends you can purchase, or you can customize them to fit your mood, combining several types of teas, such as white, green, black, ginger, cranberry, rooibos, nettleleaf, mint, rose hip, chamomile, oolong, and jasmine, to name only a few.

Coffee is rich in polyphenols. We recommend black coffee, a latte, or a cappuccino with steamed half-and-half or cream. Whether you drink red wine, dark beers, or other alcoholic beverages is completely up to you. We have our date nights when we enjoy a tasty stout or a fine red wine immensely, but we do not have alcohol daily. In our experience, limiting alcohol improves the tone of the skin and the youthful radiance of the eyes. Sometimes we cut alcohol out for months.

Marilyn's Message...

For me, vegetables are the vehicles for bringing me more anabolic foods such as lemon butter, yogurt, cheeses with plenty of antioxidant-rich herbs and spices, and unfiltered, antioxidant-rich olive oil.

On a high-carbohydrate fruit and vegetable diet, I always suffered from digestive problems due to the high amount of fiber. The Young for Life diet has put an end to any discomfort. Plenty of fat, plenty of protein, and the complement of fresh salads or warm cooked vegetables or soups feel wonderful in my body. Think about it. You're eating plenty of the foods your body needs to rebuild itself; you're a comfortably warm person, not a stiff cold person, since you're making the carbs you need and generating heat and extra calorie-burning through thermogenesis. You're not storing fat. It's your fuel, as it should be. Your skin looks great, and your nails are naturally beautiful. You're feeling far more comfortable in the clothes you love. I've spent years proving to myself that it works.

SPRITZERS

Instead of drinking alcohol, especially when it's hot, make refreshing anti-oxidant spritzers with a natural bubbly mineral water, lots of ice, and an ounce or less of cranberry, cherry, or pomegranate juice extract. For extra flavor, add the juice of half an orange and fresh mint, or slices of lime.

Here are some other ideas: Combine carbonated water with strong, fresh ginger tea to make a "ginger ale." Hot lemon water in the morning is thought to flush fats from your liver. Rinse your mouth afterward to protect the enamel of your teeth.

A teaspoon of unfiltered apple cider vinegar in water taken in the morning or any time of day, including with meals, provides potassium and may assist in the digestion of protein.

SNACKS

Since you've most likely been snacking on carbs for quite some time, your anabolic snacks will seem quite different—but soon you'll learn to love them. These are our favorites.

- An ounce of cheese, a hard-cooked egg, or a small serving of plain yogurt
- Baby mozzarella and tomato salad, or feta cheese and beets
- A handful of raw walnuts, almonds, or Brazil nuts (but be careful not to overeat nuts, because they are not easy to digest in large quantities and they are very high in calories)
- Raw vegetables dipped in almond or peanut butter

Since your primary foods on the Young for Life program are whole proteins with saturated fats and vegetables, you're following a fat loss formula no matter what you do. Except if you snack on carbs! Be sure you're not snacking because of nervousness or stress rather than of hunger. Snacking on carbs when you're in the nervous state of catabolism creates the habit of using carbs to deal with stress. This is the self-perpetuating eating disorder that leads to NDD. When you are under stress is when you most need protein, fat, and the B vitamins. Be vigilant about your snacks!

This is not a fad diet. It's a lifestyle to attain beautiful health and youthful vitality. It provides all the nutrient-dense calories your body requires for the nutrient advantage. You must eat to satiety. *Do not starve yourself!*

We ate more food and in larger portions when we started than we do now. This is fine! You'll soon realize you can eat far less at each meal when you've eaten nutrients that are abundant. This is the reality of ending nutrient deficiency disorder and enjoying the nutrient advantage.

Portion Recommendations (Per Meal)

The higher amounts are for active individuals; the lower amounts are for sedentary individuals. Amounts for snacks should be half the amounts for meals.

Proteins: 4 to 8 ounces for women; 8 to 12 ounces for men

Fats and oils: 1 to 2 tablespoons for women; 2 to 4 tablespoons for men

Fruit: For both women and men, half of a large piece of fruit, once or twice a day, before breakfast or in the afternoon; $\frac{1}{2}$ to 1 cup berries a day is an ideal anti-oxidant guideline

Nonstarchy vegetables: An unlimited quantity, raw and/or cooked, for both men and women at any meal and snack

Starchy vegetables: $\frac{1}{2}$ to 1 cup for women; 1 to 2 cups for men

---

CHAPTER **26**

Best Kitchen Equipment and Foods to Stock

WHAT YOU BUY AND HOW YOU COOK IT PLAY A KEY ROLE IN YOUR HEALTH AND YOUTHFULNESS.

I f you want to reap the benefits of the nutrient advantage, pay close attention to your cookware. A few fine pots and pans are all you need, rather than cupboards packed with old, worn-out cookware that may not be suitable for your new eating lifestyle. We find stainless steel to be the lightest and easiest cookware to use. It won't rust or lose its finish as long as you use cooking and cleaning utensils and tools designed for stainless steel. If food sticks, we simply cover the area with strong dishwasher soap or the old-fashioned, environmentally friendly natural cleanser Bon Ami, add some hot water, and allow the pot or pan to sit for a few hours. The encrusted food comes off easily, and the glossy pan remains like new.

When you're sautéing or frying, the correct cooking approach for stainless steel is to use the low-and-slow method. In other words, be careful not to heat your pans over high temperatures. Start on medium, then reduce the heat to medium-low. If you're seeking to brown the food slightly, use butter or a combination of butter and olive oil, and heat the oils slowly in the pan so they don't burn. Many foods such as fish fillets, greens, mushrooms, eggs, and onions are delicious when they're cooked in natural saturated fats, such as butter or lard, which is not a problem on this program. If you only cook with olive oil, use a generous amount so your food doesn't stick at higher temperatures.

The nonstick cookware industry grew out of a fear of fat. We didn't have these nonstick options in mass production prior to the 1960s. Most professional chefs never use nonstick, and many will tell you that low-and-slow cooking with stainless steel is cooking at its best.

Crock-Pots are great for slow cooking as well. Baked-enamel cast-iron casserole dishes, Dutch ovens, and skillets, like the products made by Le Creuset or Mario Batali, are also worth having in your kitchen. They happen to be heavy, so many people feel stainless steel is a better option, except perhaps for slow cooking in the oven. Make sure all of your enamel pots and pans are white on the inside, not red, because the red contains cadmium, which is carcinogenic.

If you use the old-fashioned cast-iron cookware that our grandmothers used and many chefs enjoy, you need to know how to care for it. The wax on new cast-iron cookware must be thoroughly removed with a brush and hot water. The cookware must be seasoned: Rub it with a thin layer of food-grade oil and heat it for at least an hour in the oven at 350°F, then wipe it clean of oil and store it where there is no humidity.

After each use, it must be cooled entirely prior to cleaning and washed thoroughly with just a small amount of soap, then dried thoroughly on a medium burner for a few minutes. Cast-iron must never be soaked. Nor can you allow cooking oils from your food to remain on skillets or pots, because that oil will quickly become rancid. You can feel it; it will be sticky, and it will spoil the flavor of the food when you use it again. In other words, cast-iron cookware is a long-lasting and inexpensive option if you care for it correctly.

The new Titanium Exclusive Cookware from Germany is worth your attention. Porcelain cookware is attractive and light, but it will break just like a porcelain plate if you drop it, and it can be costly.

YOUR YOUNG FOR LIFE SHOPPING GUIDE

Rock and I always shop for our food together. We truly enjoy sharing this responsibility. I welcome his interest and participation because he brings his own cravings to our choices. He often comes up with items I wouldn't search for or choose: a bottle of organic French wine, a low-sugar jam, such as Grandma Hoerner's organic blueberry reduced-sugar preserves. He seeks out high-quality, organic, no-stir nut butters; low-sugar, high-cacao chocolates; and a special hard salami from Germany that he loves and really appreciates when I put it in his salads. I like to ask him what he feels like eating for the next 3 or 4 days when we're at the meat counter, so my choices are as relevant to me as to him. Since we usually shop twice a week, once at Whole Foods and once at our supermarket, we plan together to buy just enough to use up everything that is perishable before we shop again. Here's what we buy:

Antioxidant-rich fruits and vegetables, and all the vegetable fruits: The polyphenol antioxidants are exhibited in the depth of color of the skins and flesh of fruits and vegetables, so eat the bright- or deep-colored apples, berries, cherries, orange-flesh melons, persimmons, and Black Mission figs, especially. Eat baby tomatoes for concentrations of lycopene. If you like grapefruit, peel it and eat the pith, which contains the bioflavonoid antioxidant. In addition, pungent, bitter, hot, and spicy flavors also indicate high antioxidant concentrations in the food. For this reason, you want to eat bitter greens, such as kale and dandelion, chile peppers of all colors, and the pungent and hot herbs, spices, and peppercorns.

Antioxidant spices and herbs: Turmeric, curry, cumin, chili, cinnamon, nutmeg, allspice, ginger, cayenne, black and colorful fresh-ground peppercorns, cardamom, bay leaves, oregano, basil, cilantro, dill, parsley, sage, rosemary, thyme, and marjoram. The pungent, hot, sour, or bitter flavors of herbs and spices signal the presence of antioxidants. Use them abundantly in your cooking, and enjoy trying our nontraditional blending of herbs and spices from different cuisines, such as Indian curry with French thyme or Italian oregano.

Celtic Sea Salt: Young for Life is not a low-salt program. Salt is a mineral you need, and it's not a good idea to avoid it. But be aware that although we use salt, if you do not like salt, you do not need to add additional salt to most of the recipes in this book. When you do want salt, Celtic Sea Salt is one product we heartily recommend. Ordinary table salt has been chemically processed to achieve its uniform crystalline structure. It doesn't include any of the trace minerals that are present in sun-dried ocean salt. Celtic Sea Salt is taken directly from seawater off the coast of Brittany, France. It's gathered and dehydrated and contains all the trace minerals your body requires.

Celtic Sea Salt will never give you the unbalanced "I'm dying of thirst" reaction that table salt and other processed "sea salts" give you, because it contains so much more than just sodium chloride and non-coagulating chemicals. It's a *health food,* and its high mineral content actually leaves your mouth feeling *lubricated,* not dry. The flavors are strong, so you need to use very little. Coarse-ground and finely ground varieties are both available.

Coffee: Coffee is a powerful antioxidant. We call it the "efficiency beverage," since we find we get far more work done after a cup of coffee. We have also noticed that drinking coffee before a workout increases our strength and endurance. Athletes often use coffee and caffeine-infused beverages as a performance enhancer. It increases calorie burning, too. Coffee releases triglycerides from your liver into your bloodstream, so, if you like, we suggest that you sometimes add cream to your coffee; you can use the fat for fuel. If you add a sweetener or consume carbs with your coffee, the fat-burning potential is lost. On our low-carb diet, we often enjoy the cream in our coffee. It helps us feel full and satisfied.

Coffee's benefits come from its polyphenols—the powerful antioxidants in foods that we can never have too much of in our diets. These are the free radical fighters that are shown to reverse aging and preserve telomeres, and they are the subject of passionate attention in biochemistry labs all over the world. Coffee definitely focuses concentration and makes you more effective.

Condiments: Look for special condiments—Dijon mustards, French mayonnaises, sauces, and salsas—that contain no sweeteners. You can also easily make the most delicious Dijon mayonnaise-style dressing (see Shrimp Salad Cleopatra on page 247) and a barbecue sauce with no sugar (page 254).

Deli-style mild pepper rings, sliced jalapeños, kalamata or sun-dried olives, sun-dried tomatoes or whole artichoke hearts in olive oil, and capers: These condiments are antioxidant rich, and they spice up a salad plate, a smoked fish brunch, or a steak.

Eggs: Organic, fertile, and free-range eggs are preferable, including those that are high in omega-3 fatty acids. The finest eggs we've found come from the free-walking hens at the Country Hen farm in Massachusetts. The shells are dark brown and hard, which are what the local New England chickens lay. (We enjoy eggs from chickens that are large and anabolic!) Their feed is pure and exceptionally high in omega-3s, and the owners are dedicated. If you find a cracked egg in your carton, they ask you to call them for a refund, but we've never seen a broken egg from the Country Hen. These eggs are available at Whole Foods, and we are able to buy them in our local supermarket.

Fresh ginger root: Use it in cooking. Or peel, chop, and boil it in water to make a pot of ginger tea, a powerful anti-inflammatory and stomach calmer that facilitates digestion and warms your whole body.

Grass-fed or organic red meats, such as beef, lamb, and buffalo and dark meat poultry and pork: Grass-fed and organic varieties of red meat can be found at Whole Foods, Fresh Market, other natural food markets, and some supermarkets and from online suppliers. We also buy organic bison, grass-fed beef, and excellent leg of lamb from Australia or New Zealand at our local supermarket. Costco sells some organic meat and poultry as well. Any organic food that is stamped "USDA Organic" will be pure meat with no filler. If you search on the Internet for any of these items, you'll find many Web-based suppliers. They often offer poultry and sausages as well.

Marilyn's Message...

During the many years that I lived on a low-protein diet, my sleep was often disrupted because I was in catabolism. Today, my favorite high-protein before-bed snack is a dish of yogurt with a tablespoon of wheat germ oil or olive oil, or a small protein shake to ensure that I have plenty of amino acids available so anabolism is in full swing. I sleep more deeply when I have had my bedtime high-protein snack; and if I've stayed up late or eaten a light dinner with a fish entrée and I'm particularly hungry, I add some cream or a little half-and-half, and 2 teaspoons of coconut oil. I recommend that you try this. Just sip it slowly and keep it small and concentrated. Too much liquid before bed can disturb a sound sleep.

Avoid low-protein, high-carb bedtime snacks during the first 3-month fat loss phase while you're breaking your carb addiction. Eating carbs will slow down the production of human growth hormone and abort glucagon, thereby thwarting fat loss. You want both these natural beauty hormones! Little Miss Muffet knew that whey and other dairy (her curds) were good for her. Long before they fell into misguided disfavor, they were rightly recognized as health foods.

Rock eats an ounce of raw or organic cheese, which he says cuts his hunger. Raw cheese is available from Organic Valley at Whole Foods, in most natural food stores, and online at farmsteadfresh.com/buy-raw-milk-cheese-online-store.html.

Green and white tea: These teas are powerful polyphenol brain tonics and belly-fat-burning drinks. The white tea comes from the baby green tea leaf, and the polyphenols it contains are even more concentrated than those in green tea, because as the leaf ages, it loses some of its polyphenol concentrations. You can drink this all day, since the caffeine is far less potent than the caffeine in coffee.

Kerrygold Irish butter, Organic Valley European-style cultured butter, and imported French, Danish, and Italian butters: Mix it up! Buy butter from many sources and soils. You'll be amazed at the difference in flavors as you sample this health food from a wide variety of farmers. Kerrygold is a pleasing choice because it's from the milk of grass-fed cows. It's available in most supermarkets and health food stores. We recommend unsalted butter because, according to chefs we know, it is fresher and has an excellent flavor; we also recommend that you avoid the commercial salt used in salted butter on your Young for Life diet. (See Celtic Sea Salt on page 220.)

Mestemacher natural whole rye bread: On the occasions that we eat bread, we make sure it's this old-fashioned, dense, chewy bread from Germany that has a delicious sourdough flavor. We prefer the wheat-free choices like natural whole rye and pumpernickel made from rye, which is the grain most often used in the healthiest German breads. When we eat grains occasionally, we prefer those we can buy from Germany and other European Union countries that have banned GMO (genetically modified) agriculture. Mestemacher whole rye bread is low in carbohydrates, because it has 6 grams of fiber in each slice. The net carbohydrate count always deducts the fiber count; thus, the net carbs per large slice equals 19 grams. One slice is enough for one sandwich, unless you're used to really filling your stomach. You can buy this bread at Whole Foods and other natural food stores or order it online from Amazon; be sure to get the natural whole rye with the green label or the pumpernickel with the blue label. Use these for Danish Open Sandwiches topped with butter and your choice of cheese, meats, smoked salmon, herring, sausage, and thin-sliced raw vegetables (see page 246). Be sure to take your vitamin C afterward to prevent AGEs, and you can also take L-Carnosine.

Nuts, seeds, and nut butters: Nuts are perishable, and their fats are prone to rancidity. So we eat more of them during the fall harvest season and winter, and less during the rest of the year. They're a cool-weather option anyway, since they're primarily high in fat and lower in protein. All nuts are good choices, but walnuts excel because they contain omega-3 fatty acids, and Brazil nuts (about six) provide the necessary selenium that is now deficient in large parts of our country's soils. Flaxseeds are also high in omega-3s; they can be stored in the refrigerator to be ground in a coffee or nut grinder and added to breading for oven-fried chicken, for example, or a protein shake. Organic peanut and almond nut butters are staples in our diet.

Organic cheeses: Organic Valley produces organic raw cheeses in sharp and mild Cheddar and Monterey Jack varieties. This company also provides the best organic buttermilk, half-and-half, sour cream,

Marilyn's Message...

Wheat and bread, particularly, are the hardest food addictions to break. We waited 3 months before we allowed grain back into our lives, because our first order of business was to break the grain habit. When you take your 72-hour carb break, before reaching for grains, have antioxidant-rich black beans. Eat them with eggs or in our Black Bean Buffalo or Turkey Chili with toppings (see page 278). Choose potatoes in their skins before grains, or try delicious Fordhook lima beans, with a net count of only 14 carbs in half a cup of soft, buttery beans. We love to eat equally delicious baby limas with fish, since fish is a lighter protein and combines better with them than heavier proteins, such as red meat, do. You'll have an easier time digesting these carbs with fish.

and cottage cheese. It is still providing the whole dairy products we recommend, in addition to low-fat options. You can also find organic cheeses at local farm stands.

Organic sheep, cow, and goat milk yogurt and kefir: There are many organic yogurts available today. Erivan yogurt, from unhomogenized milk that is pasteurized just once, is as close as you can get to the real thing. It's delicious! If you don't see it in your health food store, ask for it, or you can buy any organic plain whole milk yogurt, Greek or Bulgarian yogurt, or kefir.

Protein powders: We currently use Bluebonnet protein powders, specifically the chocolate-flavored Whey Protein Isolate and the vanilla-flavored Dual-Action Protein, which are derived from New Zealand grass-fed cows that have not been treated with antibiotics. Neither flavor is overly sweet.

Seitenbacher Muesli #21, #22, and #23: We love this German, raw, wheat-free grain, nut, and fruit cereal when we want to take a carb break and eat warm muesli with fruit and yogurt or cream prior to our workout. We didn't discover it until after we'd been on our low-carb anabolic diet for well over 2 years. Admittedly, on rare occasions it's a carb-break option that's fun and healthful. Seitenbacher makes nearly two dozen flavors, but these are the three with no added sugar beyond that in the fruit. We soak it first in hot water to soften it, drain it, and most often add cream or half-and-half and a scoop of chocolate or vanilla Bluebonnet protein powder. We sit and savor this lovely breakfast with a hot cup of coffee and Segovia playing in the background. Then an hour later at the gym, we're cookin' with energy, feeling great, fueled for anabolism and muscle shaping!

Unfiltered extra-virgin olive oil: Unfiltered olive oil was the first olive oil in the world, produced in present-day Israel by the Canaanites in 4500 BC. We recommend this type of oil for its high polyphenol antioxidant content. The flavor is strong, spicy, and delicious. Mass-produced olive oils are typically filtered, which reduces the potency of the antioxidants and the flavor. Buy extra-virgin olive oil even if you can't find the unfiltered option. Any other product is most likely a blend of olive oil and lesser-quality oils.

Virgin coconut oil and unsweetened coconut milk: Coconut is rich in the medium-chain fatty acids, which act like fat-burning cheerleaders in your body, inviting your fat cells to release fats for fuel. If you take a spoonful of coconut oil before exercising, it will burn as fuel during your workout and will also call up your own fat cells to burn along with it.

Wild-caught salmon and other fish and seafood: We enjoy all the fish we eat more if it's wild caught. We feel wild-caught fish has better flavor and texture. The bright orange color of wild salmon comes from its natural diet of shellfish, insects, and sea plants. The color of farmed salmon flesh is gray, so the farmers add coloring to the flesh to turn it a palatable orange. Atlantic salmon is nearly all farm raised because the wild fishing industries in this area were mismanaged and the wild fish populations were depleted. However, Pacific salmon, which has been better managed, is abundant. Canned, wild-caught salmon from Crown Prince is also available, so look for it in your supermarket and health food store. We eat fish twice a week: wild salmon once and another variety of fish, such as wild flounder, Dover sole, or halibut as a second seafood meal. We often have shrimp or crab in a salad for lunch in the summer.

Don't panic over organic: When shopping for vegetables, just as when shopping for animal proteins and fats, we don't panic over organic, and neither should you. Let's keep this unnecessary stressor out of our lives. The benefits of fruits and vegetables outweigh the risk of pesticide exposure, and commercial produce, especially when it is fresh, local, and in season, is far better than no produce at all, and sometimes better than organic produce that has traveled a long way in the heat and appears to be overly handled or worn out.

To reduce your commercial pesticide exposure, you can soak your fruits and vegetables in a solution of 1 tablespoon white vinegar mixed in 1 quart water. Plenty of residues will lift off the skins and leaves. Rinse well in a colander before eating. In addition, make organic fruit choices based on the following lists from the Environmental Working Group. The EWG's rankings will help you to understand which fruits and vegetables are the most contaminated with pesticides, thus helping you prioritize which to buy organic.

Commercial Fruits and Vegetables Highest in Pesticides (Try to Buy Organic)

1. Apples
2. Celery
3. Sweet bell peppers
4. Peaches
5. Strawberries
6. Nectarines (imported)
7. Grapes
8. Spinach
9. Lettuce
10. Cucumbers
11. Blueberries (domestic)
12. Potatoes
13. Green beans
14. Kale
15. Swiss chard
16. Tomatoes (our addition)

Commercial Fruits and Vegetables Lowest in Pesticides (Try to Buy Fresh and Local)

1. Onions
2. Sweet corn (update: corn is the most promiscuous cross-pollinator, so it is likely to be a GMO crop)
3. Pineapples
4. Avocados
5. Cabbage
6. Sweet peas
7. Asparagus
8. Mangoes
9. Eggplant
10. Kiwifruit
11. Cantaloupe (domestic)
12. Sweet potatoes
13. Grapefruit
14. Watermelons
15. Mushrooms

CHAPTER 27

Healthy Meals from Our Kitchen

TRY THE MEALS AND SNACKS WE LOVE TO POWER YOUR JOURNEY TOWARD A LEANER, MORE ENERGETIC, AND HAPPIER BODY.

I n this chapter, we suggest meals that will help to fuel your body for an active life. These are recipes we use, and we love them. We're not suggesting that you have to make all the recipes right away. But to help you dive in, we've chosen many that are basic, and they will give you ideas. The simplest of the breakfasts and lunches also make great snacks, and are indicated as such. The slightly more involved meals make great lunches and light suppers.

Just as important as what you eat is how you eat. Let's review some eating strategies that will help you to feel satisfied without overeating.

More important even than limiting the quantity of food is eating slowly. You need to do this to give your body a chance to register the calories you're consuming. As you eat whole protein and fat, you'll be surprised by how fast you fill up! You want to eat just enough and be sure to stop when your body signals that you don't need more. Then comes the fat burning, as the combination of protein and fat speeds up your metabolism and the fat-burning hormone glucagon kicks in. This is the natural process you're seeking that defines the anabolic way of living. You are becoming a fat burner.

Eat consciously, chew every bite until it's liquid so there is less burden on digestion, relax into positive thoughts, *enjoy your food,* and pay attention to the internal sensation that tells you that you have consumed sufficient nutrients and can stop eating now.

You won't feel the same effect from eating processed carbohydrates and sugar, because the minute you start, you've shut down glucagon and turned on insulin for fat storing. When you eat sugars, you fail to answer your body's search for the essential fat and protein building blocks of cellular repair, so your body doesn't feel satisfied. You have the sensation that you're still hungry, and you eat more. You can easily overeat, and all those calories can be stored as fat as they spike your blood sugar and set the natural emergency in motion to remove sugar from your blood and into fat storage as quickly as possible.

Fat and protein will fill you up! Be sure that your meals and snacks contain these nutrients because they're the secret to your success in dropping many pounds of fat over the next 3 months at the same time that you're shaping increasingly visible muscle tone. Fat and protein are the essential and ideal nutrients for steady and safe fat loss. The idea is to eat just enough to keep anabolism going. It may take some time to figure out how much is right for you at each meal, so you can always have a snack if you've eaten too little. And you can always eat a little less at the next meal if you realize you've eaten too much. We mastered this question of amounts by leaving excess food on our plates the minute we had the "I'm full!" feeling. There is no need to clean your plate. As you progress, you'll quickly learn how to adjust your servings to better suit your needs.

And don't forget the first tip we offered in Chapter 25: Drink a glass of water before you sit down to eat and then sip hot green tea, wine, or more water with your meal. Water will help fill you up and answer your body's need for digestive juices in your stomach.

Below you will find a collection of recipes for breakfasts, lunches, and dinners that you can make over the next 3 months during the fat-loss phase of this program. We have provided examples of the kinds of meals we eat for carb breaks as you follow our carbohydrate addiction–breaking diet. Some are very simple and quick to prepare; others include more detailed ingredient lists and instructions. We hope you enjoy them. And we hope they inspire you to create your own healthy family favorites to fuel your active lives.

We've both personally researched and experienced nearly every eating lifestyle that's out there—from water to juice fasting, raw food and wheat grass, the vegan diet, the spiritual diet, the gourmet vegetarian diet, lacto-ovo vegetarianism, and even the Atkins diet. Our Young for Life diet wins hands down!

This program is designed to nourish your body for a longer, more creative, active, and healthier life. Bon appétit!

FAVORITE BREAKFASTS

The seasons will determine the types of foods you eat for breakfast. In the warmest weather, you may not feel the need for as much fat as you do in cold weather. From our personal experience with eating heavier in the wintertime, the thermogenic effect is very real. In the hot summer, we eat lighter in the morning but make sure to get enough protein by drinking protein shakes. A creamy, cold protein shake often appeals to us as an ideal anabolic choice for breakfast, lunch, or an afternoon or postworkout meal. However, we make sure we add enough cream and a tablespoon of coconut oil to ensure a balanced protein and fat ratio. We also have protein shakes for a snack, for lunch, or even before bed, so we sleep deeply and remain in anabolism.

Young for Life Protein Shake

Protein powders are everywhere, and everyone has a favorite. We find that New Zealand microfiltered whey proteins made from the milk of grass-fed cows are fast acting and the most easily absorbed. In this microfiltered form especially, they are more digestible and will readily supply the full spectrum and high concentrations of the branched-chain amino acids in the right proportions necessary for more muscle tone before or after a workout. Microfiltered whey is absorbed directly into the muscle in about 30 minutes. It stimulates glutathione, so you receive a tremendous natural antioxidant benefit; it also stimulates the immune system and is used to nourish those who have difficulty eating during chemotherapy because it promotes muscle sparing and prevents accelerated sarcopenia.

To make the protein shake a full meal that will last longer and keep anabolism going, you can use the dual-action formula that is a combination of fast-acting microfiltered whey and slower-acting casein or whole milk protein. If we're having a light shake first thing in the morning to be followed shortly by breakfast, we simply blend the powder in 8 ounces of coconut water or purified water. A shake that is balanced in protein and fat and will keep us going until lunch will contain:

1	cup unsweetened coconut milk or milk of your choice
1	scoop protein powder (27 g protein)
½	cup fresh blueberries or frozen wild blueberries or strawberries (optional)
1	tablespoon heavy cream (6 g fat)
½-1	tablespoon coconut oil for fat burning
2-3	teaspoons peanut or almond butter (optional)

In a blender, combine all the ingredients and blend until smooth. Do not overblend or too much air will be added to the liquid and it'll be too filling.

Sometimes we skip the berries and substitute ½ cup cold coffee for some of the liquid and 1 tablespoon Dutch processed cocoa. Yummy! The fat brings satiety, so you're not immediately hungry. One scoop of protein powder is plenty per shake. Refer to the Shopping Guide for our favorite New Zealand protein powders (see page 224).

Makes 1 serving

Yogurt and Berries

When yogurt is the mainstay of your meal, be certain that it's whole yogurt, if you can find it. The low-fat dogma has so hijacked our food supply that whole, full-fat yogurt is often no longer even on the supermarket shelves. You want plain yogurt as well. Otherwise, you're eating too much sugar. You'll need from ½ to 1 cup yogurt with ½ to 1 cup berries to feel the satiation of adequate nutrition. If you find that this meal doesn't "stick to your ribs" long enough, eat the larger quantity of yogurt and, for a protein boost, stir in a few tablespoons of whey protein powder.

Marilyn's Message...
A MORNING GUIDELINE

I wake up in the morning and I want liquid and something juicy. I recommend drinking plenty of water. Twice a week, I drink warm lemon water to flush both the liver and the gall bladder, adding the juice of half a small lemon to a glass of water that is warm but not boiling. I've been using this cleansing trick for decades, and it's served me well, so I encourage you to try it. This is also when I eat some low-sugar fruit: half a peeled and sliced grapefruit, an apple, or a dish of blueberries. At this point, I'm completely hydrated and ready for some isotonics before I bathe and dress. Then I'm on to making our anabolic breakfast.

Although theoretically it's ideal to buy seasonal produce from small local or organic farms, it's not possible for everyone all the time. "Sometimes the veggies frozen right after harvest have retained more nutrients than those fresh veggies that have taken forever to get to your plate," says nutritionist Janet Brill, PhD, RD. I heartily agree!

Soft-Cooked or Hard-Cooked Eggs Topped with Whole Yogurt or Cottage Cheese

An egg-and-dairy breakfast takes advantage of the two most anabolic protein choices.

2 eggs
½ cup whole plain yogurt or cottage cheese
Fine Celtic Sea Salt
Ground black pepper

1. Put the eggs and enough water to cover them in a small covered saucepan. Bring the water to a boil over medium-high heat. Reduce the heat to medium so that the water continues to simmer, not boil. Simmer for 4 minutes for soft-cooked eggs and 8 minutes for hard-cooked eggs.

2. Remove the cooked eggs immediately from the water and cool under cold running water until you can handle them. Tap the eggs on the sides to crack them and scoop the soft yolks and firm whites out with a teaspoon into your breakfast bowl.

3. Top the warm eggs with the yogurt or cottage cheese. The contrasting textures, temperatures, and flavors are delicious.

4. Season to taste with salt and pepper.

Try green ginger tea with this kind of breakfast; it will make you feel flawless.

Makes 1 serving

Variation: Add some hot steamed greens, such as spinach or chopped red or green Swiss chard, cooked for 5 minutes or until soft. You can also top the dish with chopped seeded cucumber or diced tomato. This works as a great snack or lunch as well.

Poached Salmon with Breakfast Salad

You probably don't want your salmon to be dry, so the idea is not to overcook it. The ideal doneness is an opaque center indicating medium-rare to medium because the fish will cook slightly after it's removed from the heat. Make the salad while the salmon is poaching. This is a perfect morning meal with piping hot green tea.

Salmon

3	quarts water
3	bay leaves
2	(6-ounce) salmon fillets
1	teaspoon Celtic Sea Salt
1	teaspoon black peppercorns
1	large handful fresh parsley
	Lemon juice

Dressing

3	tablespoons unfiltered extra-virgin olive oil
1	tablespoon lime juice
$\frac{1}{8}$-$\frac{1}{4}$	teaspoon Celtic Sea Salt
	Ground black pepper

Salad

3	cups mâche, baby spinach, arugula, spring mix, or other baby greens of your choice
$\frac{1}{2}$	ruby red grapefruit, peeled and cut into segments
$\frac{1}{4}$	cup raw walnut pieces
$\frac{1}{4}$	cup pepitas (pumpkin seeds)
$\frac{1}{4}$	cup pitted Niçoise or kalamata olives
1	tablespoon whole plain yogurt mixed with 1 tablespoon water

1. *To make the salmon:* Bring the poaching water to a boil in a medium stockpot with the bay leaves. Boil for 15 minutes uncovered to reduce. Add the salmon and reduce the heat to a medium simmer. Simmer the fillets for 8 to 10 minutes, testing with a fork for desired doneness. Remove the salmon from the poaching liquid; plate; and add the salt and pepper, parsley, and plenty of fresh squeezed lemon juice. Serve immediately.

2. *To make the dressing:* Whisk all the dressing ingredients in a bowl large enough to hold the salad.

3. *To make the salad:* Combine all the salad ingredients in the bowl with the dressing.

4. Plate the salad with the hot salmon, just removed from the poaching liquid. Drizzle the salad with the thinned yogurt.

Makes 2 servings

HOW TO BAKE BACON

When you need a quantity of bacon rather than just a few strips, this is the ideal method. Preheat the oven to 350°F. Place the bacon slices on an ovenproof rack set over a large baking sheet. Bake for 20 to 30 minutes, depending on how crispy you like your bacon. Drain the bacon on paper towels and reserve the cooled drippings in a jar at room temperature for other cooking uses, such as sautéing vegetables, especially leafy greens. Drippings can be used as the first oil to choose when you are making a curried or spicy vegetable, black bean, or beef and vegetable soup.

HOW TO BAKE EGGS

It's so easy and so delicious! You'll need small, shallow, individual, ovenproof baking dishes. Preheat your oven to 325°F. Butter each baking dish. Gently break 2 or 3 eggs into each dish. Spoon 1 tablespoon cream over the eggs to keep the whites and yolks shiny and moist. Decorate and please both your eye and your palate with two or three yummies such as crumbled bacon or sausage, sliced cooked shrimp, finely chopped arugula or spinach, grated Swiss or crumbled feta cheese, minced green onions, and/or diced sundried or cherry tomatoes. Bake for 12 to 13 minutes, and serve piping hot. The variations you can make are limitless!

Rock's Arizona Scrambled Eggs and Chorizo

  1   tablespoon butter
  1   chorizo sausage
2-3   eggs
  2   tablespoons cream

1. Melt the butter in a preheated pan over medium-low heat.

2. Squeeze the sausage out of its casing and into the melted butter. Sauté the chorizo, breaking it into pieces, until it's thoroughly cooked.

3. Lightly whisk the eggs in a bowl and pour over the chorizo. Scramble the eggs with the cream until they set.

4. Enjoy this break from tradition with coffee and half-and-half.

Poached or Fried Eggs with Turkey Sausage and Parmesan Broccoli

3   turkey sausage links
2   cups broccoli florets, cut into 3-inch lengths
2   tablespoons butter
3   eggs
2   tablespoons grated Parmesan cheese

1. Grill the sausages.

2. When the sausages are almost fully browned, bring water to a boil in a small saucepan and blanch the broccoli for about 2 minutes. Drain well in a colander.

3. While the broccoli is blanching, heat 1 tablespoon butter in a skillet, break the eggs into the butter, and fry sunny-side up. You can cover the skillet just briefly to help the yolks set.

4. Spoon the broccoli onto 2 breakfast plates. Toss with the remaining 1 tablespoon of butter and the Parmesan. Arrange the eggs and sausages alongside. This also makes a terrific lunch or light supper.

Makes 2 servings

HOW TO POACH EGGS

1. In a medium saucepan, bring at least 5 inches of water and 1 teaspoon of apple cider vinegar to a boil.

2. Gently crack open 2 eggs and drop them from the shell into the saucepan when the water is at a slow rolling boil. The eggs will sink and then begin to rise to the top.

3. Poaching takes only 2 minutes. When the whites are set, transfer the eggs to a plate with a slotted spoon.

Marilyn's Message . . .
ABOUT WORKING WITH EGGS

Eggs have a special quality. As with bananas, their edible portion is neatly sealed in a shell with a tight inner membrane to keep out the air. You know how when you peel a banana and let it sit, it will ultimately oxidize and turn brown? In the same way, you don't want to abuse the sanctity of the nutrients in eggs by exposing them to the air for too long or beating so much air into them that they begin to oxidize rapidly. Wait to crack open your eggs until you're ready to use them. And refrain from beating them up. Use a whisk and beat gently and cook immediately to keep the nutrient-dense yolk from oxidizing. You'll find the gently treated egg has a fresher flavor. This is a fine point, learned from a great friend, Armand Ducellier, a chef in Avignon, France, where I was attending summer school during my junior year in college.

Another note: You'll see in these recipes that I almost always add some variety of leafy green or other vegetable to an egg breakfast. I want the additional nutrients! The iron and calcium in the greens are better assimilated in the presence of fat or if there is a high–vitamin C nutrient accompanying the meal. The inclusion of spinach, arugula, chard, or any other green you like is always optional, but for me, it is almost always a rule. I also like how colorful the meal becomes when greens are present with the eggs. Zucchini works very well, too.

Quick All-American Breakfast

1-2   slices bacon per person
1-2   eggs per person
      Pinch of fine or coarse Celtic Sea Salt (optional, since bacon is salty)
      Ground black pepper
1-2   tablespoons butter

1. Fry the bacon in a skillet until golden and just slightly crispy on both sides. Remove it from the skillet and place it on paper towels to drain. (It will continue to cook.)

2. Whisk the eggs briefly and season with salt and pepper. Gently scramble in some bacon drippings or butter over low heat or fry according to the directions given below. When set, spoon the eggs onto plates and top with bacon. Of course, hot coffee with half-and-half would be completely appropriate.

Makes 2 servings

HOW TO FRY EGGS IN A STAINLESS STEEL SKILLET

The stainless steel skillet is the perfect equipment for frying. Here's the secret on how to use it.

1. Put the butter in the skillet just as it begins to warm. Never put butter in a hot skillet. It will burn and you'll have to throw it out.

2. Start the skillet over *medium-low* heat, not high, because high heat is not friendly to stainless steel. As the butter melts, immediately turn the heat down to low.

3. Break each egg with a quick jolt from a sharp knife against the shell, open, and drop into the melted butter.

4. Let the eggs set slowly and keep them from sticking by running your spatula around the edges. You can let them cook slowly, sunny-side up, or make a nice even circle around each one so it's easier to turn them for eggs over easy.

Variation: Sprinkle grated Cheddar cheese over fried eggs for additional flavor and high biological value nutrients. Cover the skillet with a lid for just a few minutes to melt the cheese. Garnish with slices of fresh avocado.

British-Style Eggs and Smoked Kippers

The Brits enjoy their kippers, especially with eggs for breakfast. This is a great fish option, since kippers are tiny, and the smaller the fish, the healthier they are, because they eat low on the food chain and don't devour quantities of smaller fish that have already gathered mercury, PCBs, and other contaminants in widespread feeding. We love them smoked. There is practically no fishy flavor. We rinse them gently after removing them from the can, because we want buttery eggs to be the center of the plate and not soaked in fish oil.

You can fry or scramble your eggs for this yummy breakfast or lunch for a change of pace that may be a whole new experience. (It's even better if you add frozen petit peas to the scrambling eggs.) Kippers are a light protein, containing no saturated fat, so they may not fill you up as much as bacon or sausage. But they're rich in vitamin D and omega-3 fatty acids, so we recommend them highly as a good-mood food. To feel satisfied with kippers as a complement to eggs, you may want to cook your eggs in butter or lard to add the saturated fats that kippers lack.

1	can smoked kippers, drained, rinsed, and divided in 2 portions
3-4	eggs
½	teaspoon Celtic Sea Salt
1-2	tablespoons butter
½	cup frozen petit peas (optional)

1. Place the kippers on 2 breakfast plates.

2. Crack the eggs in a prep bowl and sprinkle with salt. Gently whisk just to break them up.

3. Melt the butter in an already heating stainless steel skillet and pour the eggs in as soon as the butter is melted. Stir in the peas, if using. Gently scramble the eggs until they begin to set, keeping the pan on low heat to prevent sticking.

4. Arrange the eggs on plates alongside the kippers. Enjoy with Earl Grey or English Breakfast tea or coffee.

Makes 2 servings

Poached or Fried Eggs and Sausage on Spinach

This meal will keep you full and satisfied. You can have the eggs any way you like: poached, scrambled, sunny-side up in butter, or over easy. The sausages can be natural pork, turkey, or chicken.

2	large handfuls fresh, raw baby spinach per person
1–2	sausage patties per person
1–2	eggs per person
3	Campari tomatoes, quartered
1	heaping tablespoon crumbled feta cheese per person

1. Arrange the spinach on a breakfast plate.

2. Grill or brown the sausages until brown on all sides, according to package directions. (If you're using fresh sausages, squeeze them out of the casings, form into 2" patties, and cook in a skillet until browned.)

3. Poach the eggs in boiling water until set and rising to the top, or fry them in butter.

4. Gently lift the poached eggs from the water with a slotted spoon (or use a spatula to remove the fried eggs from the skillet) and place them on top of the spinach.

5. Surround the eggs with sliced sausage and the tomato quarters and top with the feta.

Makes 2 servings

Feta Cheese, Tomato, Artichoke, and Spinach Scrambler

2　tablespoons butter, divided
1　tablespoon extra-virgin olive oil
4　canned baby artichoke hearts, well drained and quartered
4　cups fresh baby spinach
4　eggs
2　ounces soft feta cheese
½　teaspoon turmeric
　　Pinch of red-pepper flakes
½　cup quartered Campari tomatoes

1. In a skillet over medium heat, melt 1 tablespoon of the butter, then add the oil. Sauté the artichokes until heated through. Remove from the skillet and set aside.

2. Add the remaining 1 tablespoon of butter to the skillet and sauté the spinach until it's bright green and slightly wilted.

3. Lightly whisk the eggs in a bowl. Add the cheese, turmeric, and red-pepper flakes. Return the artichokes to the skillet. Pour the egg mixture over the spinach and artichokes.

4. Toss in the tomatoes and gently scramble until the eggs are set. Sprinkle with a pinch of salt, if desired, but remember that feta is salty. Enjoy this dish with hot green tea or coffee.

Makes 2 servings

Smoked Salmon Benedict with Crème Fraîche

2	cups baby arugula
1	large beefsteak tomato, sliced
4	ounces wild-caught smoked salmon
3-4	eggs
2	teaspoons capers
1½	tablespoons crème fraîche or sour cream
1	tablespoon balsamic vinegar (optional)

Divide and arrange the arugula on 2 breakfast plates. Top with the tomato slices. Layer slices of salmon on the tomato. Poach 1 to 2 eggs per person, drain on a slotted spoon, and place them on the salmon. Sprinkle with capers and top with crème fraîche. Drizzle with vinegar, if desired. Add a latte or pomegranate green tea and you're set.

Makes 2 servings

Huevos Rancheros

1	can (14 ounces) unsalted refried black beans
1	tablespoon butter
3	eggs
¼-½	cup green chili or moderately spicy tomato salsa
	Grated jack or pepper jack cheese

1. Warm the beans over low heat in a small saucepan, stirring to prevent sticking.

2. Melt the butter in a medium skillet over a medium heat and fry the eggs sunny-side up. You may need to lower the heat slightly as the eggs cook and cover them briefly to set the yolks.

3. Spoon the beans onto 2 breakfast plates and top with the eggs.

4. Spoon the salsa over the eggs and top with the cheese. Serve with hot coffee or green tea.

Makes 2 servings

Steak Chili with a Cheddar Cheese Scrambler

You may have leftover steak on occasion, and cold steak the next day isn't as appealing as it was the night before when it was steaming hot and juicy. We turn it into a quick chili for breakfast or brunch.

1	tablespoon extra-virgin olive oil
6	ounces leftover steak, diced
½	cup canned diced tomatoes
1	teaspoon chili powder
3	eggs
1	cup chopped arugula or baby spinach
¼	teaspoon turmeric
	Pinch of salt
	Pinch of ground black pepper
1	tablespoon butter
¼	cup grated Cheddar cheese

1. Heat the oil in a medium skillet over medium heat. Add the steak, tomatoes, and chili powder. Mix well and cook *just* until heated through to keep the steak from getting tough. Remove the skillet from the heat.

2. In a bowl, gently whisk the eggs, arugula or spinach, turmeric, salt, and pepper.

3. Heat a skillet to medium as you melt the butter. Pour the egg mixture into the skillet. Stir gently with a wooden spoon as the eggs set.

4. Spoon the chili onto plates and top with the eggs. Sprinkle with the cheese.

Makes 2 servings

Bacon and Broccoli Frittata

A nice brunch with a Basic Dijon Green Salad (page 249), frittatas can be served warm or at room temperature. This meal can be made in advance and refrigerated, then warmed in the oven at 300°F for 20 minutes when you're ready to serve it.

4	slices bacon
6	eggs
½	cup shredded Swiss or sharp Cheddar cheese
1	cup small-curd cottage cheese
¼	teaspoon oregano
1	cup small steamed broccoli florets, long stems removed

1. Preheat the oven to 350°F.

2. In a dry skillet over low heat, fry the bacon until crispy but not burned. Lift the bacon from the drippings with tongs and crumble it onto paper towels. Reserve 1 tablespoon of the drippings, and pour the rest into a jar when slightly cooled for future use.

3. In a bowl, whisk the eggs. Stir in the crumbled bacon and the cheeses and mix to distribute evenly. Rub the oregano between your fingers and add to the mixture. Mix gently to combine.

4. Heat the skillet with the reserved 1 tablespoon of drippings to medium. Add the egg mixture. Arrange the broccoli evenly throughout and reduce the heat to medium-low. Let the frittata cook until the sides slightly begin to pull away from the skillet, approximately 10 minutes. Bake in the preheated oven for 30 minutes. The frittata will be puffed, and the center will appear set, not runny. Cool on a rack before cutting.

Makes 4-6 servings

Variation: You can substitute 1 cup of cooked baby shrimp for the bacon.

FAVORITE CARB-BREAK BREAKFASTS

Banana Cream Quick Oatmeal

Are you craving something sweet? A hot dessert-like breakfast just might do the trick. For athletes, if you're eating this early in the day, the addition of the whey before your workout will make this a hearty, high-protein, body-sculpting meal. Dust with cinnamon from high above each bowl to bring in that spicy antioxidant benefit.

Banana Cream

1	banana, diced
1	tablespoon coconut oil
1	teaspoon vanilla
¼	teaspoon cardamom or nutmeg
¼	cup half-and-half

Oatmeal

1	cup oatmeal, quick, rolled, or whole
1¾	cups water or unsweetened coconut milk
	Pinch of Celtic Sea Salt
1	scoop vanilla microfiltered whey (optional)
¼	cup half-and-half or to taste

1. *To make the banana cream:* Put all the ingredients in a small saucepan. Stir over low heat until creamy and slightly thickened.

2. *To make the oatmeal:* Prepare the oats according to package directions. When the oats are ready, stir in the banana cream mixture and the salt. Stir in the whey, if desired.

3. Spoon into 2 cereal bowls and dust with cinnamon to taste.

Makes 2 servings

Danish Open Sandwich

Toast Mestemacher natural rye bread or pumpernickel and spread with butter. Add enough sliced raw or organic cheese, Genoa salami or Black Forest ham to feel your taste buds working, and, if you wish, some thinly sliced cucumber.

Great with coffee or green tea, this is a good carb-break breakfast or lunch. Be sure to take your vitamin C after any meal that mixes carbs and proteins (and/or L-Carnosine) to prevent AGEs from forming.

Smoked Salmon with Caviar and Blini

Arrange small slices of fine smoked salmon on a warm blini (a Russian buckwheat pancake). Add small dollops of caviar, grated hard-cooked eggs, chopped red or white onion, and sliced cucumbers.

Enjoy with a Bloody Mary—virgin or otherwise.

Muesli with Nuts and Fruit

You may want to keep fat burning going by having more protein than carbs in this bowl, so measure about ½ cup muesli for women and 1 cup for men. Pour warmed unsweetened coconut water or coconut milk over the muesli and let it soften for 5 minutes. Stir in 1 scoop protein powder for women and 2 scoops for men. Add coconut milk to taste and half a chopped banana, if desired, plus a generous handful of blueberries.

FAVORITE LUNCHES

Shrimp Salad Cleopatra

Quick Dijon Mayonnaise

1	heaping teaspoon Dijon mustard
1	very fresh egg yolk
	Pinches of Celtic Sea Salt
1	teaspoon fresh lemon juice
1	teaspoon water
¼	cup extra-virgin olive oil

Shrimp Salad

2	cups boiled, peeled, and deveined shrimp
¼	cup shaved Parmesan cheese
4	cups shredded organic romaine lettuce or mixed baby greens
¼	thinly sliced radishes (for antioxidant value, color, and flavor)

1. *To make the Dijon mayonnaise:* Put the mustard, egg yolk, salt, lemon juice, and water in your blender or food processor. Begin blending on medium speed, and then slowly drizzle the oil into the mixture to make a thick and creamy emulsion.

2. Place a generous dollop of fresh mayonnaise in your salad bowl.

3. *To make the shrimp salad:* Add the shrimp, Parmesan, greens, and radishes to the dressing. Toss well. Enjoy with iced or hot green tea or coffee or your favorite spritzer.

Makes 2 servings

Caprese Salad

Mozzarella cheese is exceptionally low in salt and high in the precious conjugated linoleic acids. This salad is so fresh and pretty. After tossing, spoon the colorful ingredients into individual shallow salad bowls. For a more robust meal in the winter, you can include pâté or top with slivers of salami. Pâtés are a good way to eat the nutrient-dense organ meats in gourmet form.

8   ounces baby mozzarella cheese, drained
     Whole heirloom baby grape tomatoes of all colors and sizes or sliced Campari tomatoes
     Handful of pitted, oil-cured olives
     Extra-virgin olive oil for ample drizzling
¼   cup fresh basil, snipped into slivers, or ½ teaspoon dried
     Drizzle of balsamic vinegar
     Pinch of fine Celtic Sea Salt
     Ground black pepper
     Imported artisan pâté or hard salami (optional)

1. Toss the mozzarella, tomatoes, olives, oil, and basil in a bowl.

2. Dress them to taste with the vinegar, salt, and pepper. Add the pâté or salami, if desired.

Italian Cobb Salad

A basic green salad forms the foundation of this meal. Highly versatile, a green salad complements any anabolic entrée. We even eat this Cobb Salad version for breakfast.

Basic Dijon Green Salad

2-3	tablespoons extra-virgin olive oil
1	tablespoon lemon juice
1	teaspoon Dijon mustard
4-6	cups fresh, tender-leaf lettuce, such as hydroponic or living lettuce
	Pinch of Celtic Sea Salt
	Pinch of ground black pepper

Italian Add-Ins

2	ounces fontina cheese, cubed
8	basil leaves, chopped
¼	pound prosciutto, sliced thin
¼	pound Genoa salami, sliced thin
4	canned baby artichoke hearts, drained and quartered
10	grape tomatoes

1. In a salad bowl, whisk the oil with the lemon juice and mustard until creamy.

2. Toss the lettuce gently with dressing, adding just a little salt, since mustard is salty. Add pepper sparingly because it may drown out the delicate flavors of the salad.

3. Now add the Italian ingredients that make this salad unusual, tossing gently to distribute them evenly.

Makes 3-4 servings

Easy Blended Salad with Avocado, Yogurt, and Salsa

If you have "salad fatigue," nothing is easier than this solution, which allows you to include all of your juicy seeded "veggie fruits" and leafy greens in a delicious drink. The combination of vegetables is completely up to you, but don't include carrots unless you have a Vitamix blender. You can experiment with the amounts of any of the following. Just make sure there are enough juicy choices to create a soupy consistency. This blended salad is an easy way to introduce more raw vegetables into your diet. Eat it for breakfast, a light lunch, or a pick-me-up snack.

Salad

2	Campari or 6 cherry tomatoes
½	red bell pepper
½	sliced, unpeeled cucumber
	Juice of ¼ lemon or lime
1	handful of parsley leaves
1	handful of baby spinach or arugula or 2 leaves romaine
½	Belgian endive
1	large rib celery
1	clove garlic (or more to taste) or 1 slice red onion
¼	teaspoon Celtic Sea Salt
	Pinch of cayenne pepper

Garnishes

½	ripe avocado, diced or mashed
1	dollop of whole plain yogurt
¼	cup salsa, preferably spicy and organic
1-2	tablespoons unfiltered extra-virgin olive oil

Put all the salad ingredients in a blender and blend until smooth. Spoon into a mug or soup bowl, stir in avocado, and top with the yogurt, salsa, and a drizzle of olive oil.

Makes 1 serving

Chicken Salad with Shaved Parmesan

A chicken salad made from the dark meat is unusual. Feel free to substitute white meat if you prefer.

¼	cup whole plain yogurt
¼	cup organic mayonnaise
1	clove garlic, pressed
¼–½	cup finely chopped celery
½	cup shaved Parmesan cheese
2	store-bought or leftover roasted chicken leg and thigh quarters
	Ground black pepper
2	handfuls baby spinach, romaine, or spring salad mix
1	handful grape tomatoes
	Extra-virgin olive oil, for drizzling

1. In a prep bowl, mix the yogurt, mayonnaise, garlic, celery, and Parmesan.

2. Toss in the chicken and add a few twists of black pepper.

3. Serve on a bed of chopped baby spinach, romaine, or spring salad mix with grape tomatoes drizzled with olive oil on the side.

Makes 2 servings

Nori Cheese Rolls

2	ounces cheese, cut from a block, such as Cheddar, Gouda, provolone, or Swiss
1-2	pieces perforated nori

Cut 1"-long chunks of cheese and wrap them in the nori to accompany your vichyssoise or any other soup or salad. Or, serve on their own for a very nutritious snack.

Makes 1–2 servings

Cauliflower Vichyssoise

Make a big batch of this soup and you'll have leftovers to complement many meals. It's a refreshing cold soup in the summer. Enjoy a mug of it with the excellent Chicken Salad with Shaved Parmesan (page 251) or with Nori Cheese Rolls (page 251).

1	small cauliflower, leaves removed
2	leeks
6	cups no-salt-added chicken broth, or enough to cover the vegetables
½	cup half-and-half, cream, or whole plain yogurt (for a tangy flavor)
	Celtic Sea Salt
	Ground black pepper
	Snipped chives or scallions

1. To core the cauliflower, cut it into quarters, set each section on a flat side, and slice away the core. Now you can more easily cut the remaining pieces into small florets.

2. Remove the dark green leaves from the ends of the leeks and trim away the roots. Slice lengthwise and then slice across the stalks and place in a bowl of water to remove any sand between the leaves. Rinse well and drain.

3. In a medium saucepan, bring the broth to a boil. Add the trimmed vegetables and return to a rolling boil. Cover and simmer until the vegetables are tender, approximately 20 minutes. Allow to cool prior to blending. You can refrigerate at this time and then complete the preparation when the soup is cold, or wait about 30 minutes before proceeding.

4. Blend the soup until smooth and creamy. Add the half-and-half, cream, or yogurt and the salt and pepper to taste and mix well on low. Refrigerate for several hours, if you haven't already done so, and spoon into bowls. Garnish with chives or scallions.

Makes 4–6 servings

South of France Egg and Olive Salad

Dressing

- 3 tablespoons extra-virgin olive oil
- 1 tablespoon lemon juice
- ½ teaspoon minced garlic
- Pinch of Celtic Sea Salt

Salad

- 6 cups tender lettuce
- 1 large roasted red bell pepper, seeds removed, cut into slivers
- 1 medium Belgian endive, cut into thin lengthwise strips
- 8 green pimiento-stuffed olives or 12 pitted, oil-cured Niçoise olives
- Pinch of ground black pepper

Eggs

- 2 tablespoons butter
- 4 eggs
- ¼ cup half-and-half or cream
- 1 tablespoon fresh thyme leaves or ½ teaspoon dried
- Pinch of Celtic Sea Salt
- Tiny pinch of red-pepper flakes or dash of cayenne pepper

1. *To make the dressing:* Whisk the dressing ingredients in the bottom of your salad bowl.

2. *To make the salad:* Add the salad ingredients to the bowl and toss gently. Set aside.

3. *To make the eggs:* Heat the skillet as you melt the butter. In a bowl, gently whisk the eggs with the half-and-half or cream and season the eggs with the thyme, salt, and red pepper or cayenne pepper. Pour the egg mixture into the melted butter. Scramble lightly with a wooden spoon.

4. When the eggs are set and no longer moist, but not dry either, break them up into fluffy pieces and fold them into the salad. Toss gently to combine.

Makes 2 servings

Cheeseburger Stack

Organic cheeseburgers? Angus, grass-fed, or Kobe beef burgers? Turkey burgers, lamb burgers? All good if you like them, and easy and yummy in a tower arrangement on a multicolored salad base. This is a pretty and delicious meal for lunch or dinner. For anabolism, most women should eat a 4-to-6-ounce burger. Men should eat an 8-to-12-ounce one, depending on size and activity levels. An iced or hot tea or coffee complements this meal.

Cheeseburger

¾-1	pound ground meat
	Celtic Sea Salt
	Ground black pepper
3	cups baby romaine lettuce
½	cup thinly sliced red onion
1	cup red or green cabbage chiffonade
1	tablespoon unfiltered olive oil
	Pepper jack, provolone, or your cheese of choice
2	thick slices beefsteak tomato
	Several thin lengthwise slices kosher dill pickle

Barbecue Sauce

¼	cup whole plain yogurt
2	tablespoons tomato paste
1-2	teaspoons smoked chili powder
2	teaspoons apple cider vinegar
2	teaspoons honey
	Pinch of onion powder
	Pinch of garlic powder

1. Form the burgers into patties of a size to suit your appetite, seasoning the meat with salt and black pepper. Set aside.

2. In a bowl, combine the lettuce with the slivered peppers, red onion, and cabbage. Toss with the oil and season with salt.

3. Begin to cook the burgers. You can grill, broil, or sauté them. Top with the cheese when you turn them.

4. Spoon half of the salad onto each lunch plate. Top with the tomato and pickle slices.

5. Prepare the barbecue sauce by combining all the ingredients in a bowl. Add 1 to 3 tablespoons of water to thin the sauce.

6. Place the cooked cheeseburgers on the tomato slices. Drizzle the entire tower with sauce.

Makes 2 servings

Grilled Sausage Salad

3	grilled sausages of your choice, sliced on the diagonal
4	Roma tomatoes, sliced
¼	cup pepperoncini
¼	cup finely sliced red bell pepper
¼	cup finely sliced red onion (optional)
3	cups spring herb salad mix
	Really good unfiltered olive oil
	Fine balsamic vinegar

Toss the sausages, tomatoes, pepperoncini, pepper, and onion (if using) together in a bowl. Divide the lettuce on 2 plates and top with the sausage mixture. Drizzle with the oil and vinegar. Serve with cucumber white tea.

Makes 2 servings

Steak Salad with Artichokes

A nice weekend treat! Made with a marinated top sirloin or flank steak, this delicious salad is easy to make. If you marinate the steak for at least 3 hours, it will be tenderized. Be sure to slice it very thinly for the proper effect.

Steak and Marinade

2	tablespoons olive oil
2	tablespoons minced garlic
2	tablespoons red wine vinegar
2	teaspoons onion powder or 1 red onion, sliced
1	flank steak or top sirloin steak (1½ pounds)

Salad

2	tablespoons unfiltered extra-virgin olive oil
1	scant tablespoon balsamic vinegar
1-2	tablespoons organic mild green tomatillo salsa
½	teaspoon crushed garlic
	Pinch of red-pepper flakes
2	cups baby arugula or spinach
4	cups spring salad mix or baby romaine
½	cup torn radicchio
½	cup slivered, oil-packed sun-dried tomatoes
¼	cup slivered red onion

Artichokes

1	can (14 ounces) baby artichoke hearts, drained and quartered
1	tablespoon olive oil

1. *To make the steak and marinade:* Put the oil, garlic, vinegar, and onion or onion powder in a shallow glass dish. Place the steak in the dish and turn it to coat. Cover and refrigerate for several hours or overnight. (Prepare the salad and set it aside before grilling the steak.)

2. *To make the salad:* In a bowl, whisk together the oil, vinegar, salsa, garlic, and red-pepper flakes. Add the arugula or spinach, salad mix or romaine, radicchio, sun-dried tomatoes, and onion and set aside without tossing.

3. Remove the steak from the marinade and grill it over medium heat for 7 to 10 minutes, depending on thickness, until medium-rare or the way you like it. Grass-fed beef is more tender and more easily digested if rare.

4. Transfer the steak from the grill pan to a cutting board.

5. *To make the artichokes:* Toss into the hot pan with the oil and allow them to sauté. While the artichokes cook, thinly slice the steak.

6. Add the steak to the salad along with the hot artichokes and toss well. Adjust the seasonings. Serve in large individual salad bowls.

Makes 3-4 servings

FAVORITE CARB-BREAK LUNCH
Easy Pork or Chicken Enchiladas
This is a great way to use up leftover roast pork or chicken. Accompany it with a Basic Dijon Green Salad (page 249) with lime used in the dressing.

1	teaspoon coconut oil or lard
1	can (14 ounces) enchilada sauce
6	whole spelt tortillas
3	cups shredded roast pork or chicken
1½	cups finely chopped spinach or arugula
1	cup grated jack cheese
	Avocado slices

1. Preheat the oven to 375°F.

2. Oil the sides of a 10" x 8" baking dish so the tortillas won't stick.

3. Pour half of the enchilada sauce into the dish and coat well.

4. Fill each tortilla with ½ cup of the pork or chicken and ¼ cup of the greens. Roll tightly and place, edge side down, in the dish.

5. Pour the remaining sauce over the all enchiladas. Top with the cheese.

6. Cover loosely with parchment or foil and bake for 30 minutes, until sauce is bubbly.

7. Plate 1 or 2 enchiladas per person and garnish with avocado slices.

Makes 6 large enchiladas

FAVORITE DINNERS

Grilled Steak and French Onion Soup

The cut of meat is up to you. Filet mignon, flank steak, or any grass-fed steak will be leanest. Bone-in or deboned rib eye will be succulent with the most fat. On the bone, it will provide the greatest amount of minerals. Season with freshly ground black pepper while cooking. Add Celtic Sea Salt only after you've let the cooked steak rest for 5 minutes, because salt draws the juices out of raw meat. Slice and serve.

Quick French Onion Soup

1	large red onion, quartered and thinly sliced
2	tablespoons butter
½	cup water
1	teaspoon dried thyme or herbes de Provence
1	pint vacuum-packed onion soup
4	slices mozzarella or buffalo mozzarella

1. In a medium stainless steel skillet, sauté the onion in the butter, adding ¼ cup of the water twice to help soften the onion. When the onion is lightly browned, add the thyme or herbes de Provence and begin to heat the soup in a medium soup pot. (This is the cue to start the steaks.)

2. Add the seasoned onion to the soup, bring to a boil, and simmer for 10 minutes.

3. Spoon the soup into ovenproof bowls. Top each with 2 slices of mozzarella and place about 10 inches below the broiler for just a few minutes, taking care that the cheese melts without overly browning. At that point, the steaks have rested for a few minutes, and it's time to eat!

Makes 2 servings

French-Style Roast Leg of Lamb

The red-meat-eating population of France rates far higher than our country's in longevity. They have just as large, if not larger, a passion for lamb as they do for beef. And they make lamb exceptionally well. There's no reason to be intimidated by roasting lamb or other meats. This is an easy roast meat recipe worth making part of your repertoire.

Lamb is the most anabolic of the red meats, because it's bone-in meat and therefore mineral-rich. Without adequate minerals in your diet, you can't absorb the all-important vitamins. Lamb from New Zealand, Iceland, and Australia is exceptionally good, and the animals are largely grass fed.

One 3½-pound leg of lamb can serve a family of 4, with leftovers for delicious sandwiches (or enchiladas). If you have time prior to roasting to marinate the lamb in the wine and seasonings for a few hours, it will be even more delicious. But if not, simply follow the directions and pop it in the oven. Serve the lamb with the Cauliflower au Gratin (page 262), which can be prepared as the lamb is roasting. A Basic Dijon Green Salad (page 249) with feta cheese complements this dish.

1	leg of lamb (about 3½ pounds), trimmed
6	cloves garlic, sliced
1	cup fine red wine
½	cup extra-virgin olive oil
½	cup dried rosemary
	Celtic Sea Salt
	Ground black pepper
½–1	cup water
1½	cups beef broth

1. Rinse the lamb and pat it dry with paper towels. With the tip of a very sharp knife, cut many slits on both sides of the lamb. Insert the garlic deep into the slits.

2. Place the lamb in a roasting pan without the rack and pour the wine over it. Cover and refrigerate to marinate or continue to prepare for roasting.

3. Preheat the oven to 450°F. Slowly pour the oil over the lamb, rubbing it into the meat to be sure the entire leg is covered with wine and oil. Press the rosemary into the skin of the lamb on all sides and season with the salt and pepper.

4. Place the lamb on a roasting rack and empty and rinse the roasting pan. Return the rack (with the lamb) to the pan and roast for 20 minutes, top side down.

5. Remove the pan from the oven, turn the leg right side up, and lower the oven temperature to 425°F. Add ½ cup of the water to the pan so that the juices don't burn.

6. Return the lamb to the oven and roast for 45 minutes, checking halfway to see whether another ½ cup of water is necessary to prevent any drippings from burning. At this point, insert a meat thermometer (but do not press it against the bone) to determine the internal temperature. The lamb should be medium rare. Turn off the heat and let the lamb rest in the oven for an additional 10 minutes; it will continue to cook to medium by the time you carve it.

7. Remove the lamb and place it on a carving board or platter. Add the beef broth to the pan drippings and set the pan over medium heat. Use a wooden spatula or whisk to loosen the drippings and dissolve them in the liquid to form a rich, natural juice. Simmer over medium heat to thicken and reduce slightly. Cut thin slices from the lamb; it will be slightly crusty on the outside, medium (pink) in the center close to the bone. Plate the sliced lamb. Spoon the remaining gravy over the meat. Add a few twists of black pepper. Serve with a fine French wine.

Serves 4

HOW TO USE LEFTOVER LEG OF LAMB

Leftover lamb also makes delicious sandwiches and can be used in a main course salad with greens, feta cheese, and Greek olives. You can also slice it cold and serve with a side of Grilled Asparagus with Cucumber in Yogurt and Dill (page 264).

Cauliflower au Gratin

We recommend serving this dish with the French-Style Roast Leg of Lamb (page 260), and it can be made while the lamb is resting. Keep it warm in an uncovered baking dish in an oven set to 300°F while you slice the lamb and prepare the gravy.

4	cups water
1	teaspoon Celtic Sea Salt
1	medium cauliflower
2	tablespoons butter
½	cup half-and-half
3	ounces yellow Gouda cheese
2	ounces sharp Cheddar cheese
1	heaping teaspoon dried basil
	Ground black pepper

1. Bring the water and the Celtic Sea Salt to a boil in a medium saucepan.

2. Remove the leaves from the cauliflower and quarter it. Slice the core from each quarter and cut the quarters into bite-size pieces. You're going to cook the cauliflower until it's soft, so the shape of these does not need to be perfect.

3. Add the cauliflower to the boiling water. Return to a boil, cover, reduce the heat to medium, and boil until soft. This dish will *not* be delicious with crispy cauliflower, so boil for 10 minutes, test, and then boil longer if necessary.

4. Drain the cauliflower well in a colander and set aside. Return the pot to medium heat. Add the butter and melt with the half-and-half. Grate the cheeses directly into the pot with a flat hand grater, stir to melt the cheese, and add the reserved cauliflower.

5. Add the basil and season with pepper. (It's unlikely this dish needs more salt, since the cheeses are salty.) Mix well. This looks almost like cheesy mashed potatoes, but it has its own uniquely delicious texture and flavor.

Makes 4–6 servings

Variation: Add chopped scallions when you mix in the butter and cheeses.

Curried Cream of Broccoli Soup

This one dates back to my earliest days as a pioneer for more vegetables in our diets, yet no one ever seems to tire of it. You can use this recipe template with carrots, acorn squash, or cauliflower. If you're cooking for adults and want the soup to have more heat, add more hot curry. For children, a very light touch of curry is all you need, or you can leave it out entirely. This soup can be served chilled or hot, and it's delicious garnished with a dollop of whole plain yogurt.

1	tablespoon butter or ghee
1½	teaspoons mild curry powder
1½	teaspoons hot curry powder
1	cup chopped scallions
1	tablespoon chopped garlic
1	cup sliced celery
4	cups chopped broccoli
6	cups chicken broth
1	scant teaspoon Celtic Sea Salt
¼	cup whole plain yogurt or more to taste (optional)

1. Heat the butter or ghee until it's just short of sizzling. Add the curry powders and sauté quickly over low heat to release the pungent flavors.

2. Immediately add the scallions, garlic, celery, and broccoli and stir well. Add the broth and salt. Bring the soup to a boil, cover, and let simmer for 30 minutes. Let cool long enough so the soup is not steaming hot. (A hot soup can cause an explosion in a blender.)

3. Blend in small increments on a low speed with the blender cover slightly ajar. Set the speed to "puree" once you're sure the soup's not jumping out of the blender. Return the soup to the pot and heat gently on medium until hot. Spoon into bowls, add the yogurt and cucumber garnishes, if desired, and serve piping hot.

Makes 4–6 servings

Grilled Asparagus with Cucumber in Yogurt and Dill

This makes a great accompaniment to leftover French-Style Roast Leg of Lamb (page 260). Fresh asparagus breaks in your hands at the point between tender and fibrous. So hold each stalk and look for where it wishes to break as you bend it.

1	pound asparagus, ends trimmed
	Pinch of Celtic Sea Salt
¼	cup olive oil or melted butter
½	small hothouse cucumber, unpeeled
1	cup whole plain Greek or Bulgarian yogurt
¼	cup fresh dill or 2 teaspoons dried

1. Blanch the asparagus in boiling water with the salt for 2 minutes.

2. Remove the asparagus with tongs and pat dry, then place it on a stove-top grill pan and brush with the oil or butter. Grill until the asparagus begins to char slightly, turning frequently.

3. Grate the cucumber and mix it with the yogurt and dill. Serve it alongside the asparagus.

Makes 2 servings

Broiled Flounder with Buttered Broccoli Rabe and Gold Creamer Potatoes

Make the vegetables before broiling the fish.

2	tablespoons extra-virgin olive oil	Pinch of garlic powder
1	tablespoon butter	Pinches of herb steak seasoning
1	pound thick flounder fillets	mix
	Pinch of Celtic Sea Salt	

1. Coat a baking sheet with olive oil.

2. Place pats of butter on the flounder fillets and season the fish. Broil it 8 inches from the broiler.

3. Test for an opaque center and remove before the fish becomes flaky.

Buttered Broccoli Rabe with Feta

Broccoli rabe is a leafy broccoli plant with tiny florets and lots of delicious greens. You use almost the entire bunch, removing only the ends of the thin stalks. The flavor is mild and not too sharp. Those who love broccoli and those who love leafy greens will appreciate broccoli rabe.

1	bunch broccoli rabe	Ground black pepper
1½	tablespoons butter	Celtic Sea Salt
½	cup crumbled feta cheese	

1. Bring 2 quarts water to a boil in a large saucepan.

2. Trim the ends off the broccoli rabe stalks (about 2 inches) and chop the rest in 2-inch segments. Rinse well and add to the boiling water.

3. Return the water to a boil, cover, and simmer for 10 minutes. Drain the broccoli rabe in a colander, gently pressing out some of the water with the back of a wooden spoon.

4. Return the broccoli rabe to the saucepan. Add the butter and feta. Season the mixture with pepper and salt. Keep warm over low heat as you broil the fish and butter the golden creamers.

Buttered Golden Creamer Potatoes

Potatoes are a good complement to a light fish like flounder. Boil the potatoes in their skins prior to preparing the fish and limit the serving to ½ to ¾ cup for women and 1½ cups for men.

1	pound golden creamer potatoes, preboiled
1-2	tablespoons butter
	Celtic Sea Salt
	Ground black pepper

1. Halve the potatoes without peeling.

2. Return to the pot in which you boiled them.

3. Heat gently with the butter and season with salt and pepper. Keep warm while you broil the flounder.

Makes 2 servings, perhaps with some leftover vegetables

Spicy Meatballs in Tomato Sauce on Steamed Garlic Green Beans

Meatballs

2	pounds ground beef or bison
¼	cup tomato paste
2	eggs
¼	cup minced fresh garlic
½	cup minced dried onions
¼	cup grated Parmesan cheese
½	cup chopped fresh parsley
	Pinch of red-pepper flakes
1	teaspoon Celtic Sea Salt

Tomato Sauce

¼	cup minced garlic
1	large carrot, finely chopped
1	large red onion, finely chopped
1	can (28 ounces) whole plum tomatoes
2	cans (14.5 ounces each) diced fire-roasted tomatoes
¼	cup tomato paste
1	teaspoon dried oregano
1	teaspoon dried thyme
1	cup chopped fresh parsley
1	cup concentrated organic beef broth
¼	teaspoon red pepper flakes
½	cup sliced, pitted kalamata olives (optional)
½	cup canned artichoke hearts, quartered (optional)

Garlic Green Beans

¼	cup peeled garlic cloves
1	teaspoon Celtic Sea Salt
	Several bay leaves
1	pound fresh green beans, stems removed

1. *To make the meatballs:* Combine the ingredients in the order given and mix well by hand or with a large spoon. Form the meatballs into golf ball–size shapes and set aside.

2. *To make the sauce:* Prepare the sauce. Drop meatballs into it and simmer for approximately 20 minutes. Test for doneness and cook no more than 10 to 15 minutes. The secret to a tender meatball is this: *Do not overcook.*

3. *To make the green beans:* Bring plenty of water to boil in a medium stockpot. Add the garlic, salt, and bay leaves. Add the beans and boil for about 10 minutes, or until tender; test at around 7 minutes to determine how much longer to cook. Drain and remove the bay leaves, but you may wish to leave the garlic.

4. Plate the beans in 4 bowls and spoon the meatballs in sauce over the top. Add a dusting of Parmesan cheese, if desired. Serve with a glass of dark stout or deep red Chianti.

Note: If you're having this meal during your 72-hour carb break, you can replace the green beans with pasta. Just be careful to watch your portions so you don't overeat on carbs. Follow the meal with plenty of vitamin C to provide the electrons that balance the free radicals resulting from mixing the proteins with the grains, and also to prevent AGEs.

Makes 4 servings

Classic Oven-Roasted Chicken with Sautéed Italian Vegetables

This is a wonderful family meal. It makes a lot of food. If you are cooking for 2 people, cut the ingredient amounts in half. Or follow the amounts listed below to have leftovers to make main course salads for lunch.

4	chicken thighs
4	chicken legs
4	chicken breasts
½	cup melted butter
3	cloves garlic, pressed
1	teaspoon paprika
	Celtic Sea Salt
	Ground black pepper

1. Preheat the oven to 400°F.

2. Wash and dry the chicken and place it in a large bowl.

3. Mix the butter with the garlic and paprika and pour the mixture over the chicken, making sure to coat all the pieces.

4. Transfer the chicken to a roasting pan in a single layer, skin side up, leaving a little space between the pieces. Arrange the breasts in the middle of the dish, with the thighs next and the drumsticks closest to the sides of the dish. Season with salt and pepper.

5. Place the pan in the oven and roast for 30 minutes, then reduce the heat to 350°F and roast another 20 to 30 minutes, testing occasionally with the tip of a sharp knife. The chicken is done when the juices run clear. The skin should be crisp and golden.

Pan Gravy for Chicken

1	cup chicken broth
½	cup white wine or Marsala

1. Remove the cooked chicken from the baking pan and allow it to sit on a platter to rest, tented with foil, for 5 to 10 minutes prior to serving.

2. Meanwhile, place the roasting pan on the stove and stir the broth and wine or Marsala into the pan, loosening all the crusty pieces and juices with a spatula.

3. Heat the roasting pan over medium-high heat until the gravy reduces to the desired thickness. Spoon over the chicken and vegetables when serving.

Italian Sautéed Vegetables

2   tablespoons extra-virgin olive oil or butter
2   cloves garlic, pressed
1   red onion, sliced
2   cups zucchini rounds
2   cups yellow squash, halved lengthwise and sliced in bite-size pieces
3   Roma tomatoes, thinly sliced in lengthwise crescents
1   teaspoon dried basil or ¼ cup fresh
    Pinch of red-pepper flakes (optional)
    Celtic Sea Salt or ¼ cup sliced, pitted kalamata olives (optional)

1. Heat the oil or butter in a skillet over medium heat. Add the garlic and onion and sauté until the onion sweats.

2. Add the zucchini and squash to the skillet. Sauté over medium heat, keeping the vegetables moving. You'll see them begin to soften. You want them to be tender not crispy.

3. Add the tomatoes and cook to warm them, but do not let them turn mushy. Add the basil, red-pepper flakes, and the salt or olives, if using, and mix well. Spoon onto plates next to the chicken.

Makes 6 servings

Balsamic London Broil
with Cheesy Broccoli

A balsamic marinade gives steak an unusual flavor. Lengthy marinating is not necessary, if you don't have time. Refrigerate for 30 minutes and then proceed to grilling.

¼	cup fine balsamic vinegar
	Plenty of crushed garlic
	Fine Celtic Sea Salt
	Ground black pepper
1	flank steak or top sirloin (1-2 pounds)
2	tablespoons extra virgin olive oil

1. Mix the vinegar, garlic, salt, and pepper in a baking dish. Add the steak. Cover and refrigerate for 30 minutes, turning once about halfway through.

2. Remove the steak from the marinade and discard the liquid. Rub both sides of the steak with oil.

3. On a stovetop or an outdoor grill, sear the steak on both sides over medium heat. Cook for 4 minutes per side, so it's rare to medium-rare; well-done London broil can be tough, especially if it's grass-fed beef, which must always be cooked on the rare side to be tender. With your knife at an exaggerated diagonal, thinly slice the steak. Leftovers of steak and broccoli can be eaten for breakfast, with a Basic Dijon Green Salad (page 249).

Makes 2-4 servings

Cheesy Broccoli

Baby vegetables are the richest in antioxidants. Broccolini is therefore a healthier choice when available, especially if you see it at your local farmers' market. If you are shopping at a market with a large variety of imported cheeses, look for imported aged Swiss, which, in many cases, will be labeled as a raw cheese.

4   cups broccoli or broccolini
2   tablespoons butter
4   ounces imported aged Swiss cheese, grated

1. Trim off the lower part of the broccoli or broccolini stems and steam the upper 4 inches until it's soft and tender. Remove to serving bowl.

2. Toss with the butter and cheese.

Quick Spinach and Artichoke Side Dish

4   cups chopped frozen spinach (approximately 1 bag)
2   tablespoons butter
8   canned baby artichokes, drained and quartered
½   cup grated or shaved Parmesan cheese, crumbled feta cheese, or both for
    a rich dish that can be used as a dip for raw vegetables
    Ground black pepper

1. In a medium saucepan, bring a small amount of water to boil. Add the spinach. Cover and cook for 5 minutes, or until tender.

2. Drain the spinach in a colander and squeeze out some of the water. Set aside.

3. Melt the butter in a large skillet over medium heat. Add the artichokes, and sauté them briefly to heat through.

4. Stir the spinach into the skillet with the sautéing artichokes. Stir in the cheese, mix well, and heat through to allow the cheese to soften and become a little runny. This is so yummy with London broil or anything else as a side dish.

Makes 4–6 servings

Braised Lamb Shanks

This is a great culinary weekend adventure, especially during cold weather. Anytime you slow-cook meat on the bone, you can be sure you're making a truly healthy meal, and lamb shanks are among the best. This is already the most mineral-rich meat, and with the bones in it's even richer. It's the old-fashioned way of using *all* the good meat, which we need to resurrect. Lamb shanks are a delicacy, and while they might seem hard to prepare, the prep time is not long, and this is an easy recipe. Your butcher probably has some lamb shanks, and most supermarkets carry them. They usually come from grass-fed lambs from New Zealand or Australia, but if you see Icelandic lamb shanks, buy them! You can always freeze them until you're ready to cook them. They fill your home with the most heavenly aromas.

If the lamb shanks are average size, plan on at least one per person. So make double the amount you'll need for one meal because this dish heats up beautifully, and you'll want to have it more than once. And a man might eat two shanks.

Wine can be used in this recipe, but onion soup works just fine, too. The tomatoes, thyme, coriander, and basil bring out the flavor. No need to add much salt. This one-dish meal will cook at a low temperature—300°F for 4 to 5 hours in a covered Dutch oven.

4-6	lamb shanks
3	tablespoons extra-virgin olive oil
2	red onions, coarsely chopped
½	cup chopped or whole clove garlic
2	cups good red wine or vacuum-packed onion soup
1	can (28 ounces) whole Italian plum tomatoes with juice
2	teaspoons dried thyme
2	teaspoons dried oregano
2	teaspoons dried basil
1	teaspoon coriander
½	teaspoon turmeric
	Ground black pepper
1	pound fresh or frozen cut green beans
4	carrots, cut into bite-size chunks
½	bunch chopped Italian parsley

1. Preheat the oven to 400°F.

2. Place the lamb shanks on a rack in a roasting pan and roast for 20 minutes to seal in the juices. After 20 minutes, remove the lamb and lower the oven temperature to 350°F.

3. While the lamb is roasting, heat the oil in a large Dutch oven. Add the onions and garlic and sauté briefly to soften. Sauté the mixture for 5 minutes and stir in the wine or soup. Bring the entire mixture to a boil and cook off the alcohol for a few minutes.

4. Add the tomatoes and the herbal seasonings to the Dutch oven and mix well.

5. Add the oven-seared lamb and season with pepper. Baste with liquid from the roasting pan, cover, and place in the preheated oven.

6. Let the lamb roast slowly for 90 minutes, lowering the heat to 325°F if it seems to be browning too fast and the broth is thickening. (You may add up to 1 cup water to the Dutch oven, if this is the case.)

7. Add the green beans and the carrots. Test the tenderness of the meat and continue roasting for another 60 minutes. Test for doneness. The meat should be falling off the bones.

Makes 4-6 servings

Chicken Parmesan with Swiss Chard in a Creamy Butter-Yogurt Sauce

6	boneless chicken breasts or thighs
4	tablespoons butter
	Muir Glen organic marinara sauce
8	ounces mozzarella cheese, cut into 6 slices
¼	cup Parmesan cheese
1	bunch green or red Swiss chard
¼	cup Greek yogurt or sour cream
	Celtic Sea Salt
	Ground black pepper

1. Preheat the oven to 375°F.

2. Sauté the chicken in 3 tablespoons of the butter until brown on both sides, approximately 15 minutes.

3. Place the chicken in a shallow baking pan and roast for 20 minutes. Remove the pan from the oven, top with the marinara sauce, mozzarella, and Parmesan and return to the oven for an additional 10 minutes, or until the cheese is fully melted.

4. Steam the chard until it's brightly colored and just soft. Drain well and toss with the remaining 1 tablespoon of butter. Add the yogurt or sour cream. Season with salt and pepper.

Makes 2 servings, with leftovers

Variation: Add herbs or spices to the chard, such as ¼ teaspoon Herbes de Provence or a dash of chipotle chili powder.

Skillet No-Crust Chicken Breast "Pizza"

Make this for lunch, make it for dinner, or pull it together in 30 minutes when guests drop by unexpectedly. You need an extra-large skillet and 4 to 6 chicken breasts for guests. This recipe serves 2.

3	tablespoons extra-virgin olive oil
2	chicken breasts, rubbed with salt
8	cloves garlic, pressed
2	large handfuls of baby spinach, stems removed
½	cup roasted red and yellow bell peppers, cut into strips
½	cup slivered red onion
8	kalamata olives, pitted
½	ball mozzarella cheese, cut into strips
1	teaspoon oregano
	Ground black pepper
¼	cup Parmesan cheese
¼	cup chopped fresh basil

1. In a large skillet over medium heat, heat the oil. Add the salted chicken breasts. Immediately add the garlic and sauté, turning quickly to brown both sides and then cooking for 5 minutes on each side.

2. Top and encircle the chicken breasts with spinach, roasted peppers, onion, and olives and arrange the mozzarella evenly on top. Sprinkle with oregano and dust with black pepper. Top with the Parmesan. Cover and cook for 10 minutes. Uncover and sprinkle with basil.

Makes 2 servings

Variation: Pinches of red-pepper flakes on top of the mozzarella are a great option for a spicier pizza.

Roast Pork Tenderloin Stuffed with Spinach and Feta Cheese

1-1½   pounds pork tenderloin
  ½   cup crumbled feta cheese
      Several handfuls of fresh spinach, finely chopped
      Blended herb seasoning of thyme, black pepper, and sage
      Chipotle chili seasoning with a barbecue flavor (optional)

1. Preheat the oven to 350°F. Slice the pork down the center, but do not cut it all the way through. Add the feta, spinach, and seasonings and close the pork over the stuffing.

2. Cut 2"-wide strips from a roll of foil. Fold each lengthwise as a tie and wrap 3 or 4 around the pork to hold it closed. You can do the same thing with cooking string. The point is to tie the pork tightly.

3. Place the pork on a rack and roast for 30 minutes. Cut into ½" slices and serve with buttered yellow beans and Euro Salad (see below).

Makes 4 servings

Euro Salad

Anytime you want a European classic, try this quick and delicious fresh salad, which we really like. The greens should be tender, like mâche, a fine farm-stand Bibb, or a living lettuce. The dressing is a simple lemon vinaigrette.

4-6   cups tender salad greens
  3   tablespoons extra-virgin olive oil (unfiltered, if possible)
  1   tablespoon lemon juice
      Fine Celtic Sea Salt

In a prep bowl, whisk the oil, lemon juice, and salt. Add the greens and toss gently but thoroughly to avoid breaking the tender leaves.

Makes 2 servings

Orange Roughy Thai Cioppino

This is an easy and creative Thai soup meal that's so tasty! The magical combination of the fish, bok choy, and spring onions in a coconut-lime broth becomes artful at the end as you toss in the bright red fresh tomatoes.

3	cups chicken broth
2	teaspoons minced garlic
½	teaspoon turmeric
1	teaspoon mild or hot curry powder
2	teaspoons Thai green curry paste
1	sweet onion, sliced
1	bunch scallions or spring onions, sliced diagonally
3	cups sliced bok choy
2	orange roughy or snapper fillets
	Pinch of Celtic Sea Salt
4	Campari tomatoes, quartered
1	cup coconut milk
½	cup chopped fresh basil
2-3	tablespoons lime juice
	Unfiltered extra-virgin olive oil (optional)

1. In a shallow soup pot or wok, bring the broth to a simmer.

2. Add the garlic, turmeric, curry powder, curry paste, onion, scallions, bok choy, fish, and salt.

3. Simmer on low for 5 to 7 minutes. Stir in the tomatoes, coconut milk, basil, and lime juice and gently increase the temperature, but do not boil.

4. Spoon into large shallow soup bowls. Drizzle with oil, if desired. Serve with finely sliced cucumbers marinated in rice vinegar.

Makes 2 servings

Black Bean Buffalo or Turkey Chili

Some like it hot, some not, so moderate your chili powder accordingly. This is a great meal anytime you're hiking or engaging in other cardiovascular activity or 2 hours before or after a workout. Have it within 3 hours of sweating, during what is called the *anabolic window,* when your body is asking both for the amino acids and for the carbs for your muscle glycogen. Make a large quantity to have leftovers on hand. This keeps well in the refrigerator for 4 days, or it can be frozen.

2	tablespoons hot chili powder
2	teaspoons ground cumin
1	teaspoon smoked paprika or chipotle blend
3	pounds ground buffalo (bison) or turkey
2	tablespoons virgin coconut or olive oil
3	cloves garlic, crushed
1	large red onion, finely chopped
2	cans (14.5 ounces each) diced roasted tomatoes
1	quart vacuum-packed beef broth
2	tablespoons tomato paste
1	can (14.5 ounces) black beans, drained and rinsed
½	bunch fresh cilantro, chopped (optional)
	Toppings: 1 or 2 tablespoons of grated Cheddar or Colby cheese, chopped red onion, guacamole, and sour cream per serving

1. Mix the chili powder, cumin, and paprika in a small bowl. Place the ground meat in a larger bowl and sprinkle with half of the seasoning mix. Knead well and then let sit at room temperature for 30 minutes.

2. In a large Dutch oven, heat the oil over medium heat. Add the garlic and onion and sauté briefly, about 3 minutes.

3. Add the seasoned ground meat, breaking it up into pieces, and brown well for 3 minutes.

4. Add the tomatoes, broth, tomato paste, and black beans. Mix well and simmer, uncovered, until the chili begins to thicken.

5. Stir in the cilantro, if using, and continue to simmer until the liquid is reduced by about half, approximately 30 minutes total.

6. Serve hot in deep chili bowls and pass around the toppings.

Makes 8 servings

CHAPTER **28**

Isotonics

DYNAMIC MOVEMENTS FOR TOTAL-BODY
STRENGTH AND VITALITY

The Royal Canadian Air Force discovered as far back as the 1960s that performing isotonics for 10 to 12 minutes a day brings cardiovascular improvements. But that's nothing compared with what we Americans should know about these movements. President George Washington invited Baron von Steuben from Germany to train his troops in these movements so they could triumph over the British in the Revolutionary War.

Today, because of our nation's sedentary lifestyle, there has been a tragic shift in our ability to train our men and women in uniform. While exceptions do exist in highly specialized units like the Navy Seals and Green Berets, and in Marine Corps basic training, the typical soldier in the US Army no longer trains with calisthenics. Instead, soldiers have been placed on a far less demanding strength and conditioning program.

America has recently abandoned the traditional demanding workout regimen that creates the strong, anabolic body—the first prerequisite for survival in combat. Regular calisthenics are now too much for our unfit recruits, who are being turned away because the training can't bring them down to "fighting weight." The long runs, pushups, situps, leg lifts, and jumping jacks, to name only a few—which have been used since at least the Civil War in our country to create the best physically prepared soldiers in the world—are being replaced by more passive exercise such as yoga, tai chi, and Pilates.

"What we were finding was that the soldiers we're getting in today's army are not in as good shape as they used to be," said Lt. Gen. Mark Hertling, who is responsible for overseeing basic training for the US Army, in an interview with the *New York Times*. "This is not just an army issue. This is a national issue."

The new training protocol uses more stretching, core exercises versus traditional situps, agility, and whole-body fitness to reduce injury and better match the challenges of the current battle environment, says the army, but clearly it has been altered to accommodate a less fit recruit.

Isotonics are dynamic movements, as opposed to static isometric contractions. Isotonics work all the muscles in a group at once and enhance flexibility. With no requirements for equipment, or even significant space, these dynamic movements can be done just about anywhere. They require only 5 to 12 minutes at home or in the office, every other day. You can break up your sessions and do them throughout the day. You should perform these movements a minimum of 3 days a week, but you can do them more often; since you're working with only your own body weight, they should not make you sore. If you do get sore, skip a day to allow for recovery. Regular use will bring out beautiful, lean muscle definition and strength, as long as you practice it often.

Isotonics use the same techniques of breathing and focus that you learned in the isometrics section (see Chapters 5 and 6). Because isotonics are movements, they result in a powerful muscle-shaping cardio routine. Add the anabolic diet that supports this routine and you'll find it's the only art, sport, or hobby that brings out your youthful side and also improves your sex life.

We're using words like *art, sport,* and *hobby* to describe this program because if you see this as "exercise," you risk making it sound difficult, and you may fail to follow through. You want to make these routines a lifelong habit that is as crucial to your good looks and health as brushing your teeth. We use terms that signify pleasure to us. Staying in tiptop shape *is* our art, our sport, and our hobby. While we're waiting in line at the supermarket or at the airport, we're contracting our glutes or abs or squeezing an imaginary orange between our shoulder blades. This is part of our recreation. We have as much enthusiasm for this as other people have for swimming, golf, yoga, Pilates, or walking.

You can expect to see and feel a difference in only a few days; in a month, bigger changes, and in a year, you're in a different body. As you give this some time, you'll see so much change and benefit that you'll have the choice, when you're ready, to cycle in some weights at the gym or at home so that you can further strengthen and sculpt your body. Going to the gym is natural, especially when you're already in good shape. It's a nice pastime, and you don't do it every day. Give yourself a day off in between to recover and tone up when you're using weights. Do it when you feel like doing it and not when you're still sore. We go three times a week, but nothing for us is a rule. First, we recommend that you do your isotonics at home or in the office, which will keep your energy up throughout the day. Don't worry about bulking up your muscles and building size. Isotonics is about sculpting an elegant shape. It is the art of creating muscle definition, strength, and graceful flexibility.

DR. ROCK REPORTS ...

The Isotonics Routine is Marilyn's secret for keeping her body tight and youthful. She can take this routine with her anywhere. In fact, I first taught it to her while we were traveling in India in 1992, where there were no gyms. She spent a lot of time ignoring it in favor of cardio when we returned, but since 2009, she has been using it every day, along with her own yoga routine and walking. She does parts of it anytime she feels the need—more than once if she likes. She uses it at home and on the road. She hates sitting for very long in a desk chair, so I often see her up next to her desk, working out. She dresses to allow for the practice of isotonics and isometrics when we travel, whether while waiting in airports and sitting on the plane. In this way, she doesn't let 2 hours of physical inactivity pass during her waking hours.

THE THREE PRINCIPLES OF ISOTONIC EXERCISE

1. Compound Movements

Compound movements involve groups of muscles. The more muscles you bring into play in any given exercise, the more anabolic your workout and the more calories you burn. The pushup is a prime example of a compound exercise. When you do a pushup, you're working your chest, upper back, triceps, and shoulders all at once. Plus, when it's done correctly, you work your abdominal muscles as well.

2. Isotonics as Cardio

Because they are movement exercises, isotonics are a form of aerobic, or cardiovascular, exercise. You'll know this the minute you do them.

The spurts of intense effort, combined with the briefest rests (10 to 30 seconds so the muscle doesn't cool down), elevate your heart rate and cause you to breathe deeply, which sends oxygenated blood to warm all parts of your body. The harder you breathe, the more you oxygenate and the deeper you go into fat burning and the acceleration of your metabolism. If you've been sedentary, overweight, or obese and are able to perform your Isotonics Routine first thing in the morning, you'll be in fat-burning mode all day. In just minutes, you've created more benefits than you can count. But "just minutes" is only the beginning. To receive the full benefits, make the effort to use isotonics for at least 12 minutes, and up to 20 minutes, three times a week. It doesn't all have to be at one time, but if you manage to put in two or three sets of 12 minutes regularly on the days you work out, you're going to see more rapid results.

Combining isotonics with isometrics provides a more effective and efficient cardiovascular workout than a lengthy aerobic session, such as running 5 miles. In fact, any cardiovascular session exceeding 90 to 120 minutes, depending on your condition and your age, can burn all the muscle glycogen you're storing as fuel and lead you into catabolism. Think about how you feel on an elliptical trainer, stair-climber, or treadmill. There is no full range of motion in anything you're doing. The motions are unnaturally repetitive for any length of time, so you risk repetitive motion injuries to your shins and knees. You're revving your engines until you're out of fuel, but you force yourself to keep going. The net effect is muscle wasting, because you've neglected to specifically, and in a focused manner, bring the correct stimulation to your muscles.

3. Concentric versus Eccentric, or "Moving through Mud"

Typically in a weightlifting exercise, the *concentric* phase is when you raise the weight and the *eccentric* phase is when you lower the weight. Most people who work with weights believe that the movement of your hand toward your shoulder in a biceps curl is what best tones the biceps. This is a concentric movement, as you curl your arm toward your shoulder and bend your elbow. The fact is, the eccentric phase is the more effective part of the exercise. Movement of your hand toward your shoulder builds perhaps 40 percent of your biceps' potential. The reason for this is that you're shortening the muscle as you're lifting.

Eccentric movement—in this case, moving your hand away from your shoulder—is always more difficult if you do it slowly, consciously, and with focus. Do it as if you were *moving through mud* and you will recruit more muscle fibers. Focusing your attention on a slower eccentric phase is one of the secrets to stronger, well-toned muscles. Try this with pushups and you'll see remarkable results.

For the quickest and most noticeable sculpting, do 1 set of 10 reps of an isotonic movement, and then rest with an isometric exercise or two. Be dynamic, and then be static. Tone your tummy actively, and then lie down or sit in your chair and use the Blue Ribbon Ab exercise (see Chapter 6). Tone your legs actively, and then pause for a moment and squeeze those buns for 6 seconds. In other words, once you've got both isometrics and isotonics down, you can go back and forth between the two techniques. Thus, as you work out, you're never *really* idle, even while resting. You will be building toned muscles all over your body at the same time that you're raising your metabolic rate (muscles burn more calories than fat), working your heart, increasing your pulse, lowering your blood sugar, and stoking fat burning.

FOCUS AND QUIT BEFORE YOU'VE HAD ENOUGH

Just one more caution and reminder: All this movement should be done consciously. Always assume a balanced stance in your best posture, with knees slightly bent, before you begin the standing movements. Make sure your abs are tight when that's part of the instructions. If you lie down, check to feel that your position is balanced, with both hips equally on the floor. Breathe, focus your mind, respect your body as an instrument and your vehicle through life, and then take pleasure in the anabolic activity that is actually going to heighten all the pleasure in your life. This is not something you approach randomly and just throw yourself into mindlessly. *You need to have a mind-set for success.* You must focus on the results you're expecting.

As you stimulate your muscles, you overcome muscle weakness, and you can begin to say goodbye to the routinely accepted soreness in the body that plagues people who are not anabolic. Pain indicates weakness. Never forget the connection. Start slowly, work consciously, and challenge yourself further *only* when you feel yourself dissatisfied with the number of repetitions you're doing. Be hungry for more but not a glutton for punishment.

"Ouch, I'm in pain! My back hurts! My knees hurt! My wrist hurts!"

Time to strengthen your forearm, back, and abdominal muscles! Time to strengthen your thighs and calves and tone your arms! You don't want surgery, do you? If you complain too much to your doctor about pain in your body, you may end up under the knife or on drugs, when all you need is to strengthen your muscles to support and cushion your spine, hips, or knees. It's a money game, and it's based on a lack of understanding of both sarcopenia and anabolism. Work to tone your abs, glutes, and legs and make the choice to avoid back, hip, and knee replacements. You can be spry into your nineties and longer. But even if you're 70, why not be able to run up and down stairs with no problem?

As a country, we don't understand the benefit of muscularity and tone. The obvious benefit is increased strength; less obvious, but just as important, is increased joint protection. If you have a well-muscled back, you are far less likely to have back pain or postural problems than a person who is overweight, skinny-fat, or skin and bone. Muscles work against gravity and protect not only the bones but also the organs. Toning your muscles stimulates the production of synovial fluid, which cushions and protects your joints.

We have a muscle-phobic society, now more than ever, that has been conditioned over two or three generations to regard the thin, untoned body as the ideal. The male waist must now be as cinched in as the female waist. The misconception or myth is that fashion dictates this abnormal thinness, and brains are superior to brawn, as if the two don't go together. This has fractured us, because brains and brawn are *both* the evolutionary genetic model we need. These isotonic movements are the secret to preventing bulking, overcoming that "square look," cutting the definition into smooth muscle, and giving you the look of a toned fitness model.

DR. ROCK REPORTS ...

I often see people doing traditional cardio routines at the gym, working out on the bike, treadmill, stairclimber, or elliptical trainer for sometimes as much as an hour. I call this the "rat on the wheel" scenario. It's overtraining and will result in catabolism. If you're over 25, you're already in the age zone when your body is naturally wasting ¼ to ½ pound of muscle a year anyway, so you're accelerating the pace of sarcopenia by working out in long cardio sessions. After overtraining, you often try to soothe the irritability of catabolism by overeating or hitting the high-sugar, processed foods. In my own experience, when I've done too much cardio, I've found myself eating much more than usual.

NOURISHING, AND TONING YOUR CELLS AND MUSCLES

Let's take a few moments to feel the effects of isotonics with a simple exercise involving your hands and arms.

Put your hands out in front of you. Now quickly open and close them 50 times. Now close your hands into fists as hard as you can for a 6-second isometric. Tighten them with a big exhaling hiss, *S-S-S-S*.

Relax. Feel that tingling sensation in your forearms, hands, and fingers as the blood flows in? You have directed your blood's nutrients into those muscles, nerves, and bones. You're feeling the anabolic effect! It's pleasurable, isn't it? You've oxygenated and fed the cells of your hands, fingers, and arms. Imagine your whole body vibrating with this nutrient advantage.

The Isotonics Exercise Routine

YOUR PLAN FOR A LEAN AND SHAPELY BODY

The Isotonics Routine is an ideal way to begin your total-body transformation. These moves are a sample of the exercises we've used for many years. They provide a full-body workout, as well as increased flexibility and oxygenation of your cells.

We like to start with some special abdominal moves because this is an area that, for most people, needs toning. The core region of your body plays a role in nearly every movement you make in life, so it is important to strengthen it. In this routine, you are working with large muscle groups such as your legs, back, and glutes and doing isolation moves for sculpted arms and shoulders.

You have three general options for following this routine.

• **Straight routine:** You can run through the entire list of exercises, doing each move once at first. Then as you progress, you can do 2 or more sets of each move back-to-back before going on to the next exercise in the sequence.

• **Circuit training:** Using a circuit-training approach, you can run through the entire routine quickly, with little rest. Once you've completed all the exercises, rest, and then repeat the circuit once or twice more.

• **Your way:** This is your routine, after all, so you can set it up any way you like. If your strength increases and you want to do 20 reps per set, please do. Before developing your own routine, start with one of the straight routine or circuit training options; then, if there is an area of your body you really want to enhance, pull a particular move from the list and do that move again at another time during the day. It may be for your abs, legs, or shoulders. Whatever you want to perfect deserves extra attention, so feel free to use these exercises at your discretion once you've mastered them.

MANAGING YOUR MIDDLE

Oh, America's aching back and pot belly! It is a well-known fact that the distended belly is a sign of potential heart disease or colon cancer. According to the late Jack LaLanne, for every 5 pounds of weight lost, you lose an inch off your waist. Do these four isotonic ab exercises first to correct or erase poor posture, back pain, and belly fat, since these may be your signature problems. This simple yet profound set of moves is designed to help elevate your heart rate, warm and limber up your muscles, and shape, tone, and tighten your waistline. Any time you do this routine, you'll initiate fat burning. Start with 10 repetitions of each move, and work up to 3 to 5 sets of 10.

Note: You must use the hard-style breath during the first four isotonics. You cannot belly-breathe and expect the result of tighter abs. Here's how: Stand tall at the beginning of each isotonic movement, inhale deeply into your chest to cause it to expand, and feel your stomach pull in and tighten naturally, as you begin to manage your middle with hard-style breathing.

With each of these moves, you can start with 5 repetitions, and then work up to 10 as you become stronger over the coming weeks. Some people may go to 20, but there is no need to push to these higher numbers too quickly or before you're sure you're ready, because the last thing you ever want to do is overtrain, burn out, and quit. Take it slow! Always want more.

Once you've reached 10 reps, begin to slowly do 2 sets of 10, and then more. The point is to find a starting level that is right for you and then increase your activity level, without doing so much that you turn yourself off. *If you do too many, back down!* The Isotonics Routine is your life raft to youth and vitality. You must always walk away feeling refreshed and energized, not tired or overworked. As you advance and develop your strength, you may work up to doing 5 sets, so you're doing 50 reps. Any reasonable extra challenge is going to bring results. But you must build up to it or you'll overwork your body, become discouraged, and quit.

And you must take time to rest! You can do your isometrics movements every day, but the isotonics require a day off between workouts for rest. You may be working every day in the beginning as you learn the routine, and that's fine, but once you have it down and begin to increase sets and reps, even if you're doing them twice a day for 12 minutes, you'll need to take a day off between workouts. It is critical that you allow your muscles to rest and recover. It's only when you rest them that your muscles build new cells and grow toned.

Now, let's discuss the isotonics moves.

DR. ROCK REPORTS...

I'm not obsessed with having the six-pack abs that some exercise experts push as the ultimate goal. My genetics make that impossible. My abs are solid muscle. They're not visibly divided. I have a four-pack, not a six-pack, and it's made of very strong muscle because I work it hard! Marilyn has a six-pack. Some people have an eight-pack. The abs are all about genetics.

I have the genetics for arms, shoulders, back, glutes, and legs, so I'm not complaining. Your genetics may be for fabulous legs, buns, or arms—or all of these and more. A six-pack involves solely the muscle group of the abdomen called the *rectus abdominis.* The muscles in this group are the flexors that allow you to bend forward.

However, if you are suffering from back pain, you must focus on the *internal and external obliques.* These muscles run along your sides and support your spine. As you tone these, you can see that coveted indentation and you can say, "Goodbye, love handles!" If you want to flatten your abdominals to fit better into your jeans and have better posture, then you must focus on your transversus abdominis—a thin muscle sheet that connects the obliques along the front of your abs and pulls the abs in when it's toned. This is the natural Spanx that you were born with. You only need to tone it. The Blue Ribbon Ab exercise you learned in Chapter 6 as you began practicing your isometric routine is a great way to tighten and sculpt this muscle.

The four ab moves in this routine will cover all these and other muscles, too, such as the *erector spinae*—the two muscles that run from your tailbone to your neck on either side of your spine to support it. Why would anyone not want to tone those muscles? You rarely see these erectors, and yet you can't have a straight back without them. Plus, toned erectors are incredibly sexy. They are the cleavage of the back. The back cleavage deserves to become as desired as a firm derrière. Let the erectors be your six-pack, and you'll enjoy a very youthful body and a straight back into old age.

Now you are in possession of the keys to the kingdom for "managing your middle."

FOUR GREAT ISOTONIC EXERCISES FOR YOUR ABS

1. Light My Fire

This first isotonic is actually our favorite warmup. But until you're familiar with it, warm up for a minute or two by marching in place to prepare your muscles and avoid injury. Light My Fire uses many muscles, so it's an extremely effective warm-up. Start off slowly and pace yourself as you heat up and become more flexible. This is a basic move, but 2 or 3 sets of 10 will have you breathing deeply and triggering fat burning. We do this one before breakfast, on an empty stomach. It's like oiling the whole body to keep it young and to remove any stiffness that makes you feel old.

How to do it:

• Start this exercise with your feet about shoulder-width apart. Stand tall and unlock your knees. Reach to the sky with your hands clasped, as if you were holding an imaginary ax, and pull your stomach up and in toward your spine.

• Reaching up high, inhale and come forward in a controlled motion and "chop" between your legs. You're moving more slowly, through mud, as you chop downward. As you exhale slowly—through the mouth, if that's most comfortable—contract your stomach tightly and reach as far as you can with your clasped hands between your ankles.

• Inhale on your way back up and come up slightly more quickly.

• Do this for 10 repetitions your first time; notice how much harder you're breathing for that coveted oxygenated glow.

Know Your Abdominal Muscles

• **Transversus abdominis:** The thin sheet of muscles running horizontally across your abs and under your skin that holds everything flat when toned

• **Rectus abdominis:** The six-pack muscle group that runs vertically from breast bone to pubic bone

• **Internal and external obliques:** Two layers of muscles along your sides

• **Erector spinae:** Two muscles that run along the spine and support your erect posture

---

2. The Windmill

This exercise is great for flattening your abs as well as working your spine and massaging your internal organs—your kidneys, stomach, and intestines.

How to do it:

- Stand with your feet about double shoulder-width apart. Hold your arms straight out from your sides, parallel to the floor.
- Bend your knees slightly and use hard-style breathing. Inhale into your chest, expanding your rib cage and pulling your stomach in tightly, keeping it pulled in even as you continue to breathe deeply.
- Now, begin to bend forward and twist to the right as you reach down to touch your right foot with your left hand. Then, remaining in the bent-forward position with abs tight, twist to the left and touch your left foot with your right hand, keeping your arms outstretched and taut, not limp, at all times.
- Repeat twisting side to side for a count of 20 reps, 10 per side.

3. Apple Picking

A great move for lengthening the spine and working the abs.

How to do it:

- Stand tall with your feet shoulder-width apart. Inhale hard, expanding your chest and pulling your stomach in tightly. Unlock your knees, keeping them slightly bent.
- Reach high above your head with your right arm, reaching slightly to the right, as if reaching for an apple in a tree.
- At the same time, extend your left leg out to the side for balance, placing only the inside edge of your big toe on the floor, pointing your toe as far away from you as is comfortable, with your heel in the air. It helps to do this exercise while watching yourself in the mirror. It's a graceful movement.
- Stabilize yourself comfortably in this position, then inhale and lower your right elbow, raise your left knee, and crunch them together on a diagonal line. Exhale at the crunch and really pull your stomach in. This one is easy if you breathe through your mouth.
- Do 10 reps on your right side, then do 10 reps using your left arm to reach and the inside edge of your right big toe to point.

4. Twist and Shout

Like Apple Picking, Twist and Shout is a tremendous exercise for flattening your abs and toning those love handles because it tightens the internal and external obliques along your sides. It's mandatory to inhale into the chest and keep your abs pulled in while doing this because you're also working the thin transversus abdominis muscles across your belly that keep your abs flat. (If you want flat, you must let your body know by holding those abs tight! Think *tightly wrapped in plastic wrap.*) But you continue to breathe deeply because your hardstyle inhalations and exhalations are coming from your chest.

The obliques are involved in twisting movements, and you *want* to strengthen them; they are the most important of your core muscles for strengthening your back, specifically the deep muscles that support the lower back.

How to do it:

• Stand tall with your feet shoulder-width apart. Inhale and fill your lungs, expanding your chest, holding your abs in tightly. Unlock your knees. Stretch your arms out to the sides, parallel to the floor.

• Twist your upper body slowly and consciously from one side to the other, going full range so you feel the contraction *on the sides* as you twist. This is the area where you focus your mind, but allow your eyes to follow the lead hand so your entire upper body is twisting. Your upper body can twist so much that your other hand will come into view, making it the new lead hand as you twist the other way.

• Do the twist at a medium tempo, and turn as far to one side as you do the other. This is not so much a momentum movement as a strong twist for the obliques; you should feel them working. Rotate—don't fling or swing—your outstretched arms from side to side. If you follow your fingertips with your eyes, you'll also exercise and relax your eye muscles for better vision, according to the Bates Method for better eyesight.

• Perform at least 1 set of 20 twists, 10 per side. This move will strengthen your back and bolster the nerves that feed your organs. After doing 1 set of these, if you wish, do 1 or 2 more during your workout day; any more can create a sore back from repetitive motion disorder. It's the quality, not the quantity, of the movement, and your focus, that will bring truly rapid results.

DR. ROCK'S PEP TALK...

The way you exercise is a metaphor for the way you live life. Put your all into it and your body will show you that there is nothing you can't accomplish. The approach you take toward the Isotonics Routine is as much about will-power and discipline as it is about the actual training. As you proceed, let this be your mantra: "From maximum challenge, I reap maximum results."

Nothing cures boredom in a workout like the fun of an additional challenge—provided, of course, that you condition yourself by working up to your challenges at a reasonable pace. I'm not saying that you should go overboard before you're in good shape (or even then), but I *am* encouraging you to learn these isotonics for managing your middle and to use them three times a week along with your isometrics, which you can use daily as often as you like. Every focused workout day will demonstrate what you can accomplish. You'll be amazed with yourself.

In Asia, your middle is known as a strong center for your chi or qi, the life energy—the power of the individual. Until recently, you would rarely see Asians with a soft middle, unless they were living in our country and embracing our diet and exercise negligence. To say your middle is your lifeline is no exaggeration.

SIX TOTAL-BODY ISOTONICS

You've worked your abs; now let's go on to six exercises that address your entire body. Unless otherwise specified, you can increase to 2 sets of 10 and then more over time. Even at this level, you'll only be spending about 10 to 12 minutes a day on the entire routine.

Be sure to rest for as long as you need to between sets. While resting, you can do an isometric, such as Elevator Lifts (see page 44), inhaling, exhaling, and tensing your glutes for 6 seconds. As we suggested above, it's always possible and helpful in toning to mix in the isometrics during the Isotonics Routine. Your time will depend at first on the shape you're in when you start. As you burn fat and become stronger, your energy will increase and your rest time may decrease. You'll also speed up as you become more familiar with the routine. On average, you may need to rest for 15 to 30 seconds between sets.

1. The Perfect Pushup

There is no better upper-body muscle-sculpting compound movement than the basic pushup. Pushups are isotonics that use almost all of the muscles in your body. You'll work your chest, shoulders, triceps, back, and abs. You'll even tense your glutes and legs. This kind of compound movement is the most effective way to stimulate overall anabolism.

Pushups can be used as cardio and muscle shaping simultaneously, and the cardiovascular benefits increase noticeably when you do more than 10 repetitions. Build up slowly: Move up to a second set of 10, and keep adding sets until you reach 5 sets of 10 reps. Our agent, Mel Berger, a highly motivated man, read this manuscript, and he was up to 200 pushups before you could say "Jack LaLanne."

How to do it:

• If floor pushups are too challenging for you at first, you can start by pushing against a wall. Stand close to a solid wall with your hands flat against it at shoulder height. Place your hands slightly wider than your shoulders. Take a big step back so that your arms are almost straight. Keep your feet flat on the floor; don't stand on your toes. Now follow the directions below, starting with the one that starts "Be a straight line," for a well-executed pushup. Before you know it, you'll be doing these on the floor.

• First and foremost, focus on your chest, not your arms. Your chest muscles will do most of the work *if* you concentrate on squeezing them to make the movement happen. Even with this focus, you will be toning your arms and the rest of your body.

• Position yourself facedown on the floor, balancing on the balls of your feet or toes, with your fingers spread and palms firmly on the floor. Your hands should be directly under your shoulders. Your body should form a straight line from head to toe. (If you are a beginner, do these on your knees first. You'll "graduate" fast to full pushups on the toes. The anabolic firming of your entire body is a benefit worth the effort.)

• *Be a straight line,* holding your abs flat and your glutes tighter than tight. Avoid sagging in the middle or allowing your bottom to arch up into the air.

• Now is when you're "moving through mud"—the eccentric part of the movement, when you recruit the greatest percentage of your muscle fibers. Inhale deeply, and exhale slowly as you bend your arms and lower your body to the floor. Take about 4 seconds for this lowering phase. This recruits more muscle fibers because you're working against greater resistance, as gravity is trying to pull you down fast. Lead with your chest, not your head or your hips. Keep your neck perfectly lined up with your head and body in one straight line. Your body should feel sleek, long, and taut, not limp. All muscles, therefore, are participating.

• At the bottom of the movement, inhale and tense your chest deliberately. Now begin the concentric phase. Push up rapidly as you straighten your arms and rise to the top of the pushup without locking your elbows.

Common Pushup Mistakes to Avoid

Looking forward: Hyperextending your neck can cause neck injuries. Keep your neck aligned with the rest of your spine from start to finish. Keep your eyes focused on the floor directly below your face, not in front of your head. Don't hang your head down, and don't pretend you're a swan. Keep a level form from head to toe.

Letting your torso droop: This is often caused by weak abdominal and back muscles. Focus on the isometric of your abdominal muscles, keeping your body in a straight line from your ankles to your shoulders. Tighten your abs and squeeze your glutes to keep yourself straight; only do as many pushups as you can with perfect form. If it's just one, that's great! Before you know it, it will be two, then four, then five and up. And this happens fast, so give it a chance.

Variations When the Basic Pushup Is Too Hard

If you find the full pushup position too difficult, then just hold your body in the up position for as many seconds as you can without lowering your body. This is one of the best isometrics, and you can gain a tremendous amount of toning from it. It's a good version of what is commonly called the plank, which is sometimes executed balancing on the forearms.

2. Stunning Thighs

Stunning Thighs is a remarkable compound movement that also firms your glutes, hamstrings, and calf muscles. It even helps to firm your abs and lower and upper back, and it strengthens your hips and knees. Some trainers call Stunning Thighs the Hindu Squat. We do a special version

DR. ROCK'S PEP TALK...

The muscle is clay. It's the mind moving the muscle that shapes the muscle. It's how much you focus your mind on the muscle you are shaping that creates the shape. When you move to weights, keep the poundage low enough so you're not flinging or relying on momentum to move them.

Rule: It's not the weight, but rather it's the conscious contraction of the muscle that makes you a successful body sculptor.

of the squat in Stunning Thighs that makes all the difference in how effective it can be. When you reach the upright position at the end of the movement, you will gently thrust your hips forward while tensing and contracting your glutes and the muscles of the pelvic floor. (It helps to do this exercise in front of a dressing mirror to perfect your form.) Your pelvic floor muscles, including your pubococcygeus muscles (PC for short), are those you squeeze to stop the flow of urine. You may be familiar with Kegel exercises, in which you squeeze the PC muscles for a few seconds per repetition. Strengthening these muscles helps both men and women experience more powerful sexual sensations. You'll gain these benefits, plus strengthen your lower back and create better posture, by adding this extra "secret" move to Stunning Thighs.

How to do it:

• Stand tall with your knees unlocked. Put your hands in front of you as if holding an invisible broomstick. Keep your arms taut to balance yourself as you lower your hips slowly to a seated position, as if there were a chair to sit on. Resisting this downward phase as you move slowly recruits more of the muscle fibers.

• In this position, keep your back erect; you should be leaning forward only slightly. Your knees should not be dramatically projecting over your feet. You only need to go down to the point where your thighs are parallel to the floor. Keep your arms taut and outstretched in front of you (unless you have lower back problems, in which case support yourself with your hands on your thighs).

• When you reach the bottom, you enter the concentric phase. Move upward as you raise your body to standing position at a slightly faster speed. At the top of the movement, with your arms outstretched at chest height, push your hips forward while tensing and contracting the glutes and the pelvic floor muscles.

• At the same time, row your arms back and squeeze an imaginary orange between your shoulder blades to enforce erect posture and build a strong back. What good are stunning thighs if you're slumping forward because of a weak back?

• Stretch your arms in front of you, and you're ready for your next repetition.

Don't worry about leaning forward if you have to when you first begin this movement. You are making the motion of sitting down, so it is natural for you to lean forward slightly; but as your thighs strengthen, you'll use them more to lower yourself, and you'll find you can keep your back straighter.

Forget about the scale and tape measure! Be more influenced by what you see when you look in the mirror. This is what a sculptor does. You'll see soon enough that your pants will be looser, and you'll be going down in dress or jean size, inch by inch, as you tone and sculpt, replacing the dead weight of fat with active, lean muscle.

When you perform Stunning Thighs, you are working many large muscle groups, making this one of the most anabolic movements of all. You're strengthening libido, raising testosterone and human growth hormone, and improving the uptake of insulin-like growth factor. These hormones keep you young and sexy, creating ongoing anabolism and repair in your body. This one isotonic should become a pivotal part of your routine. Work up to 5 sets of 10. The key is to keep your focus on the leg muscles throughout the exercise.

3. The Bun Shaper

The Bun Shaper is the antidote to the sagging backside. As a toning tactic, it gives your butt that coveted, round, high shape and lift. Because your glutes are your most powerful muscles, you must stimulate them *hard* for results. (In surveys, women report that their favorite part of the male body is the glutes. This sexy body part raises women's heart rates like exercising on a treadmill. So guys, tighten those glutes and save some lives!)

Marilyn's Message...

Ah! The Bun Shaper! There's simply no better secret for lifting the derriere. I used to do 150 at a time, but that caused a burnout I regretted. Now, after paying the "burnout price" of watching my buns begin to go south, I suggest that you work up to 5 sets of 10 if you want stellar results. But take your time, starting with 1 set of 10. You only want to do enough so that you always love the Bun Shaper. At this point in my routine, I usually do 2 sets of 25. It's natural to increase your reps as you become stronger. You'll inevitably outgrow the 1 set of 10! Congratulations on starting! You'll be seeing buns you never thought were possible sooner than you can believe.

Note: A trick for faster results is to use the Elevator Lifts isometric exercise (see page 44) in your final one or two repetitions. Inhale, exhale, and squeeze those buns for 6 seconds before lowering your legs to the floor.

How to do it:

• Find a padded chair or bar stool that is strong and sturdy enough to hold you as you stretch your torso across the seat, facedown. Place your hands on the floor to brace yourself or hold on to the legs of the chair. Your stomach and hips should be on the chair. Your chest and shoulders should be balancing off the chair to offset the weight of your legs.

• Keep your legs straight, with your toes on the floor. Inhale deeply and raise your legs above parallel, or just slightly higher. To ensure that you're not straining your lower back, use the muscles in your glutes, not your back, to perform this movement. Do not arch your back or you will make your lower back sore. Hold your legs up and squeeze the glutes for at least 6 seconds for the isometric benefit. Tighten them as hard as you can, until they shake, and keep that tension for 6 seconds while you exhale. Repeat this powerful, shaping isotonic several times or until the blood is really flowing and your backside is tingling.

4. Dangerously Classy Calves

The calf is a shock absorber for the knee, so if you are willing to develop your calves, you'll save much wear and tear on your knees. If your calves

DR. ROCK REPORTS...
The Vital Principle of Rest

Muscles are stimulated with exercise, but it is when you stop exercising that they go through the process of toning and growing. Specifically, it is during rest that significant rebuilding and repairing takes place.

Too often I've witnessed the overzealous athlete—the exercise addict who never misses a workout, runs 6 miles a day, or is on the treadmill sweating and exhausted every time I go to the gym. This is the person who goes from a 10-K to boot camp to Spinning to swimming, and then off to do hot yoga at night. This form of overtraining keeps you in catabolism, and it's actually dangerous. You may be happy because you're emaciated, with a serotonin high, but in fact, you're most likely skinny-fat, with plenty of jiggle on your abs, because this amount of exercise is bound to burn skeletal muscle. If you do too much, look in the mirror, because you will look exhausted and see signs of aging. Premature lines and wrinkles will speak to you about overdoing your exercise capacity. This is a signal to pull back.

Here is the good news about this system of anabolic exercise: It requires

---

aren't strong, you will also have foot and ankle problems later in life. And the sculpted calf, compared with a smooth, shapeless lower leg, is far more attractive, whether you're barefoot or in heels.

This move is best performed on a step or some kind of platform so you can rise up and then lower your heels below your toes for the maximum stretch and contraction. As you stretch, you recruit more muscle fibers when you rise back up on your toes. Hold on to something stable, like a banister, as you perform this movement and keep your mind on the calf muscle exclusively.

How to do it:

• Stand tall with your feet together, knees slightly flexed, the balls of your feet on the step and your heels hanging off.

• Rise up on your toes as high as you can, pause, and then slowly lower your heels until you feel the stretch in your calves. Perform you to rest. When you are beginning with only a few minutes of isometrics, it's not a problem. You can benefit, and you need the daily exercise. But once you're up to the 3-sets-of-10-to-20 range of isotonics, or you're doing 30 minutes to an hour of focused exercise, even in 10-minute segments, work out every other day. This may mean working out three times a week with a rest between each day, and then four times the next week with a rest between each day. Since you're doing this at home or in the office during short breaks, it's up to you.

An option we like is to take the weekends off. These off days and weekends are when the walking, yoga, tai chi, and other soft arts can become a part of your life. If you're older than 50, the rest time to recuperate and secrete growth hormone is even more critical. In fact, it's mandatory! It's a known fact in physiology that when you stimulate the muscle, if you keep stimulating it, you'll undermine your progress. You *must* allow it to rest and grow stronger and more toned.

People think that top bodybuilders and champions must be in the gym all the time. Actually, the pros are in and out. They go into the gym, focus their efforts, use maximum intensity, and get out. Then they put their focus on their nutrition and their rest.

20 repetitions. End your session with a calf isometric, holding for 6 seconds and squeezing your calves at the top of the movement until your calf muscles shake.

5. Beautiful Biceps

There is a secret to achieving the coveted, curvaceous appearance in your arms. Here's what makes all the difference: the position of your hand as you do the biceps curl.

This exercise employs two hand positions. First, to pop the peak (or center) of the biceps, you should position your hand as if it were holding a hammer. Create a light fist as if grasping a pencil, with your hand straight up and down. It's not a tight fist. You can see the biceps peak pop when you use this hand position.

The second position is also with a fist, but as you reach the top of the curl, you turn your fist toward the outer biceps, palm facing up. This shapes the outer head of the biceps, which emphasizes the cut between your shoulder (deltoid) and the biceps muscle. These two positions will be particularly essential when you begin to use weights to tone your arms.

How to do it:

Hammer Fist for the Peak: Stand with your feet firmly planted on the floor, knees bent slightly, abs contracted to make a strong, conscious, and focused foundation for this movement. Make two fists in front of you with your elbows lightly against your sides. Your fists are not tight, and they do not do the work. It's the tightening of the biceps muscle—specifically the peak in the center—that creates the lift.

• As you tighten the biceps of both arms, the fists begin the curling motion up toward the shoulders at the same time. Keep your fists in the hammer position—that is, palms facing in as if holding hammers; don't rotate them. Count "one-one-thousand, two-one-thousand" as your fists nearly reach your shoulders, then consciously lower both arms at the same time.

• The lowering in this case is a quicker motion because you're only tensing the biceps in the lifting of the fists. Remember, it's the tightening of the biceps that actually causes the lift, not the tightening of the fists.

• Start with 1 set of 10 and work up to doing these three times a day.

• **Rotating Fist for the Outer Head of the Biceps:** Place your left hand, palm down, firmly on top of your palm-up right fist. Begin curling your right fist toward your shoulder against the resistance provided by your left arm. As you flex this way, curl up to the count of 6.

• At the top of the curl, rotate your right fist as if the little finger were trying to touch your outer shoulder or deltoid, so that your palm faces forward. Tighten and squeeze for a 6-second isometric benefit while you hold this twist. *Do not strain.* Only hold the twist for as long as is comfortable, up to 6 seconds. The result will be a peak contraction of the outer head of the biceps, which creates the more sculpted effect.

• At the completion of the concentric curl, lower your fist without counting, rotating it back to the palm-up starting position. After completing a set with your right arm, repeat the exercise with your left arm, as detailed below.

• Use the exact same technique with your left arm, placing your right hand firmly against your left fist and curling up slowly to the count of 6,

Marilyn's Message...

Realizing the importance of going to sleep early was one of my major steps toward becoming Young for Life. The hours before midnight are your beauty sleep hours. The earlier you go to bed, the greater your chance for deep and restful sleep. This is the natural design. We only learned how to extend the day far into the night a little more than 100 years ago, with the invention of the light-bulb. Turn off the lights. Go to bed. Capture your rest to recapture your youth!

rotating your fist outward and holding for 6 seconds in an isometric contraction. Then lower your left hand as you lowered your right fist, without effort.

• Repeat this rotating fist exercise for 2 sets of 5 initially (or 1 set of 10) and slowly build up to 3 or more sets of 10 over the course of a day, rather than all at once, to prevent elbow fatigue or soreness.

• The key is to keep your mind on your biceps at all times, concentrating, not just to move randomly, without focus.

As you become stronger, you may wish to purchase a pair of dumbbells for greater resistance. Five pounds is a good starting weight for women. Men may wish to start with 10 to 20 pounds. You will then see the major benefit of these two fist positions: outstanding shape in the muscles of your arms.

6. Taut Triceps

Who's happy with floppy triceps? You only need to know what to do to put that issue behind you. You have already worked them with your pushups, so you don't necessarily have to do more. But if you want a specific triceps exercise, try this one for excellent results. It's an easy move that anyone can do.

How to do it:

• Hold your hands palms together in front of your chest as if praying. Slowly, with focus, as if you were pushing through mud, straighten and spread your arms down in opposite directions, as if you were reaching to flatten your palms against an imaginary wall behind you. Keep your arms in line with your shoulders and feel your triceps tense. Hold that tension for 6 seconds, squeezing your triceps. (For a more intense isometric, start with your palms against a wall behind you and press into the wall.)

• Return your arms to the starting position in front of your chest, with palms together. Repeat 10 times and work up to 3 sets of 10, resting between sets. These sets can be done throughout the day for faster results.

Epilogue

The healing and regeneration of the body doesn't usually happen in a vacuum. Nothing Rock and I have accomplished on our own journeys to restore our declining bodies to youth and health can be said to have happened through our mere human effort. It was our faith and our belief in something far greater than ourselves that guided us on this path to bring this message of health and healing to you. It was the deepest conviction that, with God as our partner, we could not fail, which allowed us to push forward when Rock's very life was on the line. We never quit; we never backed down. A beautiful inner guidance insisted that we succeed for *your* sake.

Now, you have the gift we believe we've been guided to share. We invite you to approach this moment in your life as a truly sacred time. It is your time to cherish the life you've been given and achieve freedom from suffering. You are not alone, just as we were not alone. And we want you to know that we are enthusiastically cheering you on toward success.

We're living in exciting times! On the cusp of a revolution! With your participation in our program, your ability to walk away from disease is rapidly gaining momentum. This information that is so groundbreaking didn't come to you randomly. You reached out for it! We wish to congratulate you for taking the significant steps to be Young for Life. What lies ahead for you is truly exciting. In our experience, there is no ceiling on regaining youth. The process is incremental. Life and your enthusiasm for living it in a strong, pain-free, and agile body and with a mind full of youthful confidence become easier and better. Nothing is sweeter at any age than the capacity to share the "young love" that accompanies this kind of rebirth.

We invite you to come to our home on the Web at marilyndiamond.com and share the story of your own journey to youth to inspire others. You'll find many resources to assist you. We'll keep you updated, because even as this book goes to press, new information became available that we are impatient to share with you. As we work together to help you achieve your goals, accept with our commitment to you, dear friend, that we love you deeply. We hope you feel with confidence how happy we are to finally be with you!

Marilyn Diamond and Dr. Rock

Resource Guide

W e encourage our readers to continue their education and health-improvement efforts to stay Young for Life. Following are sources for additional reading as well as products and publications mentioned in this book.

Recommended Reading

Yudkin, John. 1972. *Pure, White and Deadly: How Sugar is Killing Us and What We Can Do to Stop It.* New York: Penguin Books.

Rodale, Maria. 2010. *The Organic Manifesto: How Organic Gardening Can Heal our Planet, Feed the World and Keep Us Safe.* Emmaus, PA: Rodale Books.

Keith, Lierre. 2009. *The Vegetarian Myth: Food, Justice and Sustainability.* Crescent City, CA: Flashpoint Press.

Ravvnskov, MD, PhD, Uffe. 2009. *Fats and Cholesterol Are Good for You.* Sweden: GB Publishing.

Smith, Jeffrey M. 2007. *Genetic Roulette: The Documented Health Risks of Genetically Modified Food.* Portland, ME: Yes Books.

Appleton, Nancy, PhD. 2009. *Suicide by Sugar: A Startling Look at Our #1 National Addiction.* Garden City Park, NY: Square One Publishers.

Pollan, Michael. 2008. *In Defense of Food: An Eater's Manifesto.* New York: Penguin Publishing Group.

Emord, Jonathan W. 2010. *Global Censorship of Health Information: The Politics of Controlling Therapeutic Information to Protect State Sponsored Drug Monopolies.* Sentinel Press.

Price, Weston A., DDS. 2009. *Nutrition and Physical Degeneration.* Lemon Grove, CA: The Price-Pottenger Nutrition Foundation.

PREVENTION, Rodale Inc. Read by our parents before us, *Prevention* was the first publication of its kind to stress the importance of supplements, nutrition, and exercise as keys to a healthy life plan. It remains a cutting-edge health magazine and one of the best-researched consumer publications for improving one's health. We also recommend *Prevention*'s sibling magazines *Men's Health* and *Women's Health*. Marilyn's home gardening skills for years have been honed by reading *Organic Gardening*, another Rodale magazine.

SUPPLEMENTS: All of the vitamin and mineral supplements recommended in this book are available at pharmacies, grocery stores, health food stores, and nutrition stores. As we've mentioned, we take a special vitamin C formulation containing mineral cofactors in powder form. C-Youth is available for online order at marilyn diamond.com. While quality vitamin C supplements are widely available, we are champions of this original formula and the great scientists whose work contributed to its discovery and countless benefits.

IN THE KITCHEN WITH MARILYN: What are Dr. Rock and Marilyn eating today? Find out and take advantage of recipe updates, nutrition news, and additional tips to build your Nutrient Advantage at marilyndiamond.com/inthekitchenwithMarilyn.

THE LIFE EXTENSION FOUNDATION: This nonprofit organization funds research dedicated to finding scientific methods for addressing disease, aging, and premature death and reports on breakthrough nutrition, fitness, and medical news in *Life Extension Magazine*. A free 6-month membership and magazine subscription (a $29 value) are available to *Young for Life* readers at lef.org/YFL. LEF members receive free access to naturopaths, nutritionists, trainers, and other health advisors and personalized antiaging programs, plus discounts on nutritional products through the Life Extension Foundation Buyer's Club.

Acknowledgments

Here's to you, Mel Berger, our friend and agent of nearly 30 years at William Morris Endeavor Entertainment. Your unique dedication and enthusiasm triggered the record-breaking status of *Fit for Life*. How exciting that you're here with us at this time, sharing this vision, embracing these ideas, modeling the youthful dynamism, and working your magic to ensure that *Young for Life* reaches our deserving audience.

Jeff Csatari, executive editor of *Men's Health* and Rodale Books, what a tremendous honor to work with you. Thank you for grasping the importance of this message and for skillfully guiding us through the editing process to bring *Young for Life* to timely publication.

Ariel Soffer, MD, cardiologist, you and your beautiful wife, Maria, warmly welcomed Rock in your office to verify the depressing diagnosis after congestive heart failure of a shortened lifespan. During challenging times, you heard his determination to win his battle and offered good science, open-minded support, and friendship that exemplifies the excellence of your profession.

Philip Smith, an amazingly talented man, author of *Walking Through Walls*, and editor of *Life Extension Magazine*. Thank you, Philip, for your patience as we brought this manuscript to the right place at the right time to be able to receive your timely review and assistance for reaching our audience.

Lyndon Wright, the brilliant Internet expert, what a gesture of encouragement for us that you jumped on the program with so much success and added your personal commitment to spreading the word. You're a first-class creative professional!

Our dear friends: Helene Layne, associate director at Xcelerator Media Group, you read the first draft, dropped eight dress sizes without dieting, and looked closer to the age of your daughter. *Thank you!* Dr. Froukje and Jeroen Kuyper and your colleague Martje DeAntje, our gratitude for your tireless assistance in keeping our work going abroad, as leaders of the Dutch Power of Love organization. Jackie Blankenship, our beloved personal assistant in the Power of Love—accept our appreciation for reading and rereading the early drafts and for being here to assist, no matter what the need.

New friends, who expressed so much desire to be Young for Life and were willing to read the unedited manuscript prior to publication: Steve Sarno, screen writer and coproducer of *Born to Race* I and II relished his high-protein and -fat diet, ate to satiety without touching a carb, lost 50 pounds, and walked away from chronic pain in less than 7 months; Tricia Forbes, who fought her carb addiction and used the Isotonics and Isometrics to dramatically change her shape to chiseled and who looked radiantly younger in 4 months, with the only complaint being that she had to keep buying a smaller wardrobe; Kay Lorraine Caringi, who studied the manuscript thoroughly, reading and rereading for mastery. She has become a model of success, going from a middle-aged body she refused to accept through a breathtaking metamorphosis. She has defied aging, looks younger than she has in 10 years, and is bouncy and brimming with confidence.

Boundless gratitude and love to our family, Julie and Bruce Everett Schnell and Ginger Schnell for your constant and powerful prayers, family encouragement, and the wisdom of your advice.

Finally, our children, Greg and Annie Neuwirth and Lisa and Rob Lusk, thank you for your willingness to share your blessings and turn tough times into the best times. Thank you for your kind words that bolster and inspire us and the memorable gatherings you fill with love and laughter; Beau Diamond, we are so grateful for your enduring love and support and your example that no matter what life dishes out, we can stand tall and grow stronger in mind, body, and spirit; and Sathya Schnell, we honor your exemplary brilliance to excel at subjects that only 1 percent of the population can master, and we thank you for your patience and loving understanding of our effort.

The biggest hugs, smiles, and kisses to our four precious grandchildren, Max, Gus, Remy, and Miles. It is you who show us the way. You, good and beautiful people, make your Ama and Baba proud. You're the reason we wrote this book. We love you enormously. You're the reason that we made it our job to know how to be active and young for life.

Index

Underscored references indicate boxed text.

for diabetes prevention, 27
loss of, 13, 26 (*see also* Sarcopenia)
Muscle strength, increasing with
    isometrics, 30, 31
Muscle-to-fat ratio, 14
Muscle tone, benefits of, 285
Muscle wasting
    adverse effects of, 13–15
    catabolism and, 19, 24–25
    causes
        overtraining, 283, <u>286</u>
        sedentary lifestyle, 13
    compensating with anabolism, 26
    early-onset, 14
    high blood sugar linked to, 14–15
Muscularity, 285
Myoglobin, 191

N

National Library of Medicine, 7, 52, 57
NDD. *See* Nutrient Deficiency Disorder
Neck
    exercise for, 36–37
    injuries, 296
    pain, 36–37
Nervous system, B vitamins for, 73, 78–79,
    81
Neuropathy, diabetic, 14, <u>71</u>, 78
Niacin (vitamin B₃), 76–77
Nitric oxide, 51
Nori
    Nori Cheese Rolls, 251
Nursing homes, 11
Nut butter, 223
Nutrient Advantage
    B vitamins, 68–83
    described, 49
    food guide, <u>210</u>
    iodine, 84–90
    vitamin C, 58–67
    vitamin D, 91–99
    vitamin E, 50–57
Nutrient Deficiency Disorder (NDD)
    described, 3
    diagnosis of, 4
    fighting with
        anabolism, 22
        carbohydrate reduction in diet, 130,
            152

high biological value protein, 115, 119
micronutrients, 45–49
health care policy issues and, 5–9
    artifacts disguised as food, 5–6
    censorship and profits, 7–9
    Dietary Reference Intake (DRI), 6–7
Nutrients. *See also specific nutrients*
    B vitamins, 68–83
    essential, 122
    iodine, 84–90
    side benefits of, 48–49
    soil depletion of, 80, 85
    vitamin C, 58–67
    vitamin D, 91–99
    vitamin E, 50–57
Nuts
    Poached Salmon with Breakfast Salad,
        234–35
    shopping for, 223

O

Oatmeal
    Banana Cream Quick Oatmeal, 245
Obesity
    carbohydrates and, 123, 170
    Centers for Disease Control and
        Prevention goal, 5–6
    in children, 11, 14
    low-fat diet and, 149, 153
    processed food and, 5–6
    statistics on, 21
Olive oil, 225
Olives
    Caprese Salad, 248
    Italian Sautéed Vegetables, 269
    Poached Salmon with Breakfast Salad,
        234–35
    Skillet No-Crust Chicken Breast
        "Pizza," 275
    South of France Egg and Olive Salad, 253
    Tomato Sauce, 266
Onions
    Black Bean Buffalo or Turkey Chili, 278
    Braised Lamb Shanks, 272–73
    Cheeseburger Stack, 254–55
    Grilled Sausage Salad, 255
    Grilled Steak and French Onion Soup,
        259
    Italian Sautéed Vegetables, 269